PRAYERS
FROM

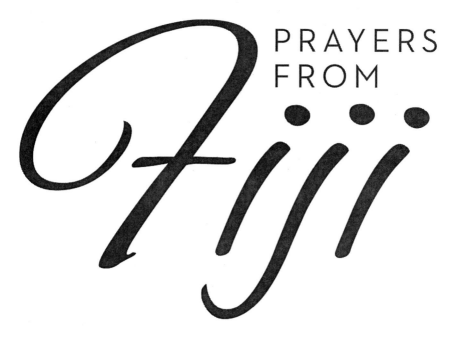

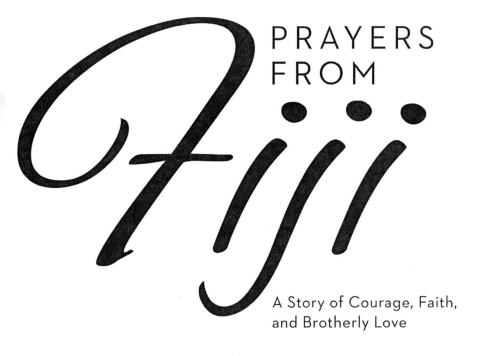

PRAYERS FROM Fiji

A Story of Courage, Faith, and Brotherly Love

Ellen Murkison

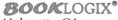**BOOK**LOGIX®
Alpharetta, GA

The medical accounts contained in this book are those of a single individual from the perspective of her immediate family and friends. These accounts are not intended to convey specific medical advice to any other individual, and they are not intended to provide recommendation for or against any specific choice in medical care.

The author has tried to recreate events, locations, and conversations from her memories of them. In some instances, in order to maintain their anonymity, the author has changed the names of individuals and places. She may also have changed some identifying characteristics and details such as physical attributes, occupations, and places of residence.

10 9 8 7 6 5 4 3 2   0 6 0 6 1 4

Printed in the United States of America

ISBN: 978-1-61005-502-4

Cover Art: Deborah Harvey Graphic Design
Cover Photography: Lori Grice Photography

CaringBridge is a registered trademark of CaringBridge, a nonprofit organization.
Facebook is a registered trademark of Facebook, Inc.
Lands' End is a registered trademark of Lands' End Direct Merchants, Inc.

♾ This paper meets the requirements of ANSI/NISO Z39.48-1992 (Permanence of Paper)

To my boys, your strength and love inspire me every day. To my husband David, I could have never made it through this experience without you. I love you all so much.

For nothing will be impossible for God.

Luke 1:37

Contents

Part One:
The Accident and Hospitalization

Part Two:
Rehabilitation and Return to Real Life

Part Three:
Lessons in Faith

Part One:

The Accident
and Hospitalization

In this portion of the book, the events are told in chronological order, beginning with the night of December 2, 2011, and ending February 7, 2012. The descriptions are of the events as I remember them. Though others may have different memories of certain events, I attempt to relay the story only from my own perspective. When using the word "we," I refer to my husband David and myself, and use the pronoun "I" when it is my personal recollection or thoughts, not a memory that he and I share collectively.

1

The Crash

We did what hundreds of American families do on a December night. We piled in Grandpa's Ford Explorer (with a third row, room enough for the six of us) and headed out to a Christmas light show at a nearby farm. It was something we had all done before, and we were looking forward to seeing the lights, the crazy inflatable snowmen, and the mock western town that the owners of the farm had created.

It was a Friday night, and my husband David, our two boys (Ben, age ten, and Brian, age seven), and I had driven down from Atlanta that afternoon to David's hometown of Statesboro in south Georgia. We'd left early in the afternoon and arrived well before dinner. Because we'd gotten to town so early, David's mom and dad suggested we could go visit the lights after we ate, and we all agreed.

This was probably the fourth or fifth trip to Statesboro we had taken since school had started, and one of the only times we'd arrived before eight or nine p.m. We had just moved to Atlanta the previous July, and were still making frequent visits back to town to see the grandparents and our friends, to attend parties and football games, and to go to our old church, St. Matthew's. It was accurate to say that I at least was quite homesick for Statesboro, and while the three-and-a-half-hour drive wasn't something to enjoy, I jumped at every chance we could go back.

Earlier that day David and I drove up to the school to collect the kids, and I remember sitting in the circular driveway waiting for them all to come out. Apparently, when they called Ben to the office he had forgotten something back in his class, so instead of them all walking out together, David allowed Brian to come out to the car first.

Do you have memories that you never forget? Snapshots of a moment of time? I very clearly remember watching Brian come bounding out of the school, down the sidewalk toward the car, and thinking, *Oh, Ellen, look at your beautiful child . . . remember this.* He was happy and excited to be called for "early dismissal" and almost bounced down the sidewalk. The bright blue sky was behind him and the sun was literally shining off his blond hair. I had a moment where I just saw him, heard that voice in my head, and thought how lucky I was to have such a great kid. He jumped in the car and the talk immediately turned to what happened at the playground, in class, etc.—the normal, everyday, after-school kind of stuff. A few minutes later David and Ben got to the car and we took off on our trip.

I didn't think a thing about that moment until later, but it would become one of the last memories I had of Brian before everything changed. I realize that was God's voice whispering to me to stop. Look up. Look at the gift of my child right in front of me. How often do we look but not actually see what is right in front of our eyes? In that moment, God blessed me with the ability to not only see but to remember, and as the events of that day unfolded, it was something that I held to when the rest of my world fell apart.

That night our family enjoyed seeing all the elaborate, bright, and fun Christmas lights, but the evening was chilly, so after walking around a bit, we headed back to the car. David's dad was driving and his mom sat in the passenger seat. David and I mirrored them, but sat in the middle row, while the boys scampered into the Explorer's third row, Ben on the left and Brian on the right, directly behind me. It was small, but for little boy legs, not a big deal to sit back there. Brian, still being seven, had his booster seat, and everyone buckled up.

It was about nine o'clock at night, I guess. We were all chatting and talking, there were at least two different conversations going on in the car while we drove down the dark two-lane country blacktop road away from the farm and back towards the town. This road was not a place any of us typically drove, and on the way out to the lights, we even second-guessed which road to turn on. You know the sensation of thinking "I'll know it when I see it" when you've been somewhere before but can't picture the exact details? For me at least, this was how I considered the route to and from this farm.

I glanced out my window, and as if in slow motion, my mind took in the headlights of a car heading toward us while at the same time I saw a stop sign intended for our road. I knew in that split second we were going to be hit, but I couldn't get a word to come out of my mouth to warn anyone. The next thing I remember is hearing a loud noise and feeling our SUV spinning. The official accident report says that our car entered the intersection just as the other vehicle drove through and we were hit on the rear right side of the vehicle, the very spot Brian was sitting. The force of the impact spun us around and eventually the SUV tipped up on its side and collided with a car waiting on the opposite side of the intersection. Even though all of this took less than a minute to occur, I have lost count of how often I have thought about that split second in time that changed our lives forever.

I never lost consciousness, and remember asking David if he was okay and hearing my father-in-law talking to us in those first few moments. I had been hanging by my seat belt, and I managed with shaking hands to undo it and get myself free. My heart was racing, I was in shock I am sure, and scared to death, yet felt compelled to keep calm. I think back and realize it was through God's grace that my mind was able to focus, and I could begin to talk with David about getting the boys out of the back. As the car was sideways, it was disorienting and difficult. Within a minute or two, the people in the car sitting on the opposite side of the intersection had gotten out to help us.

Initially, we were able to get Brian's seatbelt off him, and pull him to the middle row and then out of the car. It did not register with me in the moment that he was unconscious or that he may be seriously hurt. Ben was next to come out, and by this time other people had arrived on the scene. One man critical to the story was named Tyler, an off-duty EMT whose family owned the farm we had just visited. Though it was not his normal route, he had been traveling on that exact highway and came up on the scene. A big muscular guy, he was one of the people who lifted the car up as we tried to pull Ben out. The seatbelt was stuck, and Tyler had a pocketknife that he used to cut it off him so we could pull Ben from the car. Both of my in-laws were also safely removed from the car at this point.

Ben was hysterical, bloody, and crying. Both David and I had been able to get free of the car, and while David went to where the people had lain Brian on the ground, I stayed with Ben. He lay on the ground, crying and screaming, and I put my face down to his and tried to comfort him, not knowing if he was crying because he was injured, terrified, or both.

To say I was scared was an understatement. I felt no pain myself, but I can still feel the fear that overcame my heart in those moments. It was chaotic, dark, and loud as the people on the scene tried to help us. Because Ben was so clearly injured and bleeding, Tyler made a call to the local air evacuation helicopter EMTs and gave them instructions on how to get to the scene of the accident (several miles from the nearest town). The ambulance was also called and began making its way to the scene. In the short time it took for the helicopter and ambulance to arrive, Tyler and the EMTs had already recognized that Brian, unconscious and beginning to show signs of posturing, needed to go first, even though Tyler had initially called for the helicopter with Ben in mind. Posturing—a reflex the body takes when the brain is shutting down or injured, putting Brian in a fetal position with his arms curled up toward his chin—was a terrible sign.

I was probably twenty feet from Brian, and did not realize that he was being taken off in the helicopter at the moment it was happening. I stayed with Ben, who was by this time beginning to calm down a little but was scared that the EMTs would be giving him a shot. His fear of needles had in that moment become a centerpiece of his reaction, and even though he was hurting and bleeding, he was only concerned with not getting a shot. I remember giving Ben my attention, not realizing until later that a helicopter was taking off into the dark night sky, carrying Brian off to the trauma center at Memorial University Medical Center (Memorial) in Savannah, fifty miles away.

I was later told by the trauma doctors in Savannah that had Brian arrived even twenty minutes later than he did he would not have even survived the trip to the ER. It was God's plan for Tyler to be on that road at that exact time, because had the normal protocol happened, no helicopter would have been called until after the ambulance had arrived. But who did God see fit to be traveling that road? Someone with firsthand knowledge of not only what to do, but *who* to call to get that helicopter to the scene. That difference in time was all that it would have taken for Brian to have died that night, possibly right there on the side of that road.

The paramedics from the ambulance joined me next to Ben and put him on a stretcher. He was moved into the back of their rig, and I went with him. It was at that time I asked where Brian was and his status; the EMTs told me he had been taken to Savannah. They assessed Ben, and determined he also needed to go via helicopter to the hospital in Savannah. I immediately began to ask them if they were going to drive me to Savannah, because I *needed* to be with my children. No answer to that question came; the ambulance simply drove Ben, my father-in-law, and me to the Statesboro airport a few miles away. The airport is little more than a landing strip and a few buildings usually reserved for private planes or crop dusters. As we approached, the fear in my stomach was growing; I felt so helpless. We pulled up next to a helicopter and Ben was taken straight from the ambulance to being put on board. I wanted to go with him, but was told there was no room on board for anyone except the patient, the EMT/nurse, and the pilot.

It was horrifying, but I had no choice. Ben was crying and pleading, and I had to try to remain calm and reassure him it was going to be okay, all the while feeling sick to my stomach that it was not. The crew made me get back in the ambulance and the helicopter took off. I sat in the front seat, my father-in-law had been moved to the back of the ambulance, and the driver told me that we were headed to the ER in Statesboro probably ten minutes away. I continued to say, "I need to get to Savannah, how am I going to get to my boys?" but he couldn't say. David and my mother-in-law were being transported to the Statesboro ER at this time as well, and when we arrived at the hospital, I was brought in to see them.

They were in two separate rooms of the ER, and I remember asking my mother-in-law if we could find someone who could call one of our friends in town to bring me to Savannah. I had not brought my purse on the trip to the lights and had no money, no cell phone, and was definitely not in any mental condition to be driving myself the hour-long trip to Savannah at that point. I was able to talk with David, who was being treated for cuts on his face and checked for internal injuries, and told him I was planning to get to Savannah somehow. He was being sedated by this time, and needed to just let the doctors care for him.

Again, God clearly intervened. He had it planned that I would make it to Savannah that night, because a doctor leaving his shift at the ER came up and told me he lived in Savannah and would be able to drive me there. I decided I needed to get my purse and cell phone, but my mother-in-law did not have a key to their house. She told me to see if their neighbor was home and she could let me in. As I got in the car with this kind ER doc, I asked him if we could please take a minute to stop by my in-laws' so I could get my purse, and he agreed. We drove up their street and parked at the neighbor's (coincidentally, she was an ER nurse at that same hospital and knew the doctor, so while she gave me the key and I ran across the street, he filled her in with what details he knew of the accident). I grabbed what I needed and ran out the door, and we drove off into the night.

The doctor was calm and was trying to distract me as we drove, but my heart was racing and the sick feeling in the pit of my stomach was growing (that feeling didn't go away for what seems like months, although it was never quite as strong as that hour in the car). As he drove, I tried calling my friends Kristen and her husband Joe. Not reaching either of them, I kept trying to call their cellphones. They had been having dinner at Kristen's parents' house that evening and didn't want to interrupt dinner to answer the phone, but when they kept hearing first Kristen's then Joe's phone ring repeatedly, they realized something might be wrong. I was so relieved when Kristen called me back and I could sob to her that we were in an accident and I was on the way to Savannah and could she please come. With the grandparents already right there able to watch their kids, both Joe and Kristen immediately got in their car and made the drive to the Memorial ER where they would end up meeting me.

While I talked to them, the doctor driving me called the trauma department at Memorial to get an update for me and to tell them he was bringing the mother of the two boys who had arrived via air evac. As I finished my conversation with Kristen, I could hear him talking to the doctors, several of whom he knew personally, having worked in that ER before as well. He handed me his phone, and I heard a trauma doctor tell me at that moment, Ben had arrived and was being treated in the ER for his injuries and was going to be fine. But what he said next almost caused my heart to break right there in the car. He said Brian had suffered a severe head trauma and the doctors had already taken him into emergency surgery to remove a bleed on his brain. He made it clear, it was life threatening and there was no reassurance of any kind that it was okay. It was the first of many times that I would be given a medical prediction that Brian's life was almost over.

2

The First Night

My memories of the first few hours at the hospital are limited. When I think back to that time I can still feel the sick feeling in my stomach that accompanied waiting for them to tell me anything. I arrived at the ER at the same time as Joe and Kristen, and their presence with me that night is something I consider the most selfless act I have ever seen. The nurse called me back to the ER, and Kristen came with me, never letting go of my hand. We were brought in a small room where Ben was lying on a table. In the harsh glare of the hospital lights, he looked terrible—blood on his face, his eye bruised and red, in pain, and scared to death. It was clear he was so relieved I was there, and I held his hand and talked to him, it was a beautiful moment when at least the two of us were back together.

The staff eventually moved him upstairs to the Pediatric ICU (PICU) and he was asleep after a short bit. They told me he'd been given a lot of pain medication and sleep aids and he wouldn't be waking up anytime soon, and suggested we move out to the waiting room.

The PICU waiting room, how I came to value and loathe that room. Institutional chairs, the kind in a doctor's waiting room that can't be separated . . . vinyl seat covers . . . a vending machine . . . a TV. This was the place I awaited the doctors' news about Brian's surgery. Sitting with Joe and Kristen in a daze, totally in shock and scared to death about what was about to happen. I wondered how I got there and how this could be happening. Eventually they came to tell me Brian made it out of surgery and was being moved into the PICU. Again, Kristen held my hand and we walked through the doors so I could see him.

It is her recollection of what happened next that follows because my memory of this part of the night is so hard to capture. She said I walked in the room and before she knew what was happening I had dropped to my knees making the sign of the cross and praying for God to help my baby. What *I* remember is that he was attached to a ventilator with a tube coming out of his mouth. He was connected to an IV machine with numbers and wires and God knows what all those medicines were for. Worst of all, his head was bandaged and a giant metal spike was sticking out of it. As they explained the spike's purpose, the feeling in my stomach just got even worse. I remember trying to comprehend the information the doctor was telling me. I was like most of you reading this book. I had no background, no experience, and no knowledge about what a traumatic brain injury means. Unlike the prognosis of how Ben would be (expected to recover just fine), the prognosis on brain injuries is almost always poor, especially when they are the severity of Brian's injury. What follows is my own interpretation in layman's terms of what was told to me at that point.

The brain is just like any other part of the body. If it sustains a blow or trauma, blood and fluid rush to the site of the impact and cause it to swell (just as your ankle might swell if you break it). But unlike most other parts of the body, the brain cannot withstand excessive swelling. The skull is made of some of the hardest bone in the body, designed to protect the brain. But in this case, the skull itself would provide too small an area once his brain began to swell. The doctors knew this reaction would be coming, so they intentionally left a piece of Brian's skull out after operating on him. It was the right side of his head in the frontal area, approximately from his ear to his forehead.

Even with a piece of his skull removed, they expected the chances were very high that his brain would eventually swell until it crushed down his brainstem. At the point your brainstem is no longer functional, you are considered brain dead. The primary swelling would be occurring during the first seventy-two hours following the impact, and until the end of that time, the pressure inside his head would get higher and higher. The spike in his head measured that pressure, and the number taunted me from that moment on. Seeing it rise or fall was a sick obsession.

David and my mother-in-law, Marilyn, would eventually arrive and I joined them in the waiting room. They told me my father-in-law Gene was in critical condition as well, and had been flown to Savannah by the same helicopter that flew Brian to Memorial and was on a different floor in the ICU. David had been treated for some internal injuries at the hospital in Statesboro and he was in a lot of pain, and the medication he had been given was making him fall asleep. It was also the middle of the night by this time. My in-laws' neighbor who had lent me the key to their house had driven them, and they had been thoughtful enough to bring my suitcase so I could wash my face, take out my contacts and put on my glasses, and just try to prepare myself for what was going to happen next. I immediately went back in the PICU to be at Brian's side.

Upon hearing the doctor's initial words to me, I remember asking the nurses to please find out if the hospital had a priest on call. My dad had been praying rosaries throughout the night back in Illinois, and each time I spoke with him, he asked me to please find a priest to come and give Brian his last rites. I asked the nurses, but didn't get an answer. A little while later, when they couldn't find anyone, in desperation I asked my friend Joe to help. Without a second's hesitation, he set out. Savannah is a beautiful city, but it has many areas of high poverty and crime. The area where the hospital is located is right on the edge of some not very safe neighborhoods. Despite the risk, Joe eventually found a Catholic church and knocked on the door in the middle of the night. Father John Lyons answered that door, and before I knew it, he had arrived at the hospital.

Brian was given the sacrament of the Blessing of the Sick (also known by most as the last rites). Father John led us in prayer over Brian's bedside that night, asking God the Father and Jesus to please bring healing and wholeness back to our child. I have never

13

forgotten the comfort it brought me to at least know that Brian had received this blessing, and if he was about to leave this world, I had done what I thought was best in terms of preparing his sweet soul.

After Father John left, the night wore on. My memory of every hour after that is hazy, but I know the morning eventually came. Joe and Kristen had been able to contact many of our friends and family for us overnight, and eventually left to get a few hours' sleep in a hotel nearby. Because I had not been examined by a medical professional at the scene or at the Statesboro ER, David insisted that I go down to the ER to be checked out. It was nerve-wracking and scary to be away from the PICU; all I wanted was to get back upstairs. I thought how stupid it was for me to be downstairs being x-rayed when my son was upstairs dying! The shock and exhaustion was getting the better of me, and at one point, I just started crying. A minister from the hospital joined me in the room while I was waiting for the doctor, and I jaggedly told her what was happening. I don't remember exactly what scripture she shared with me that morning, but I do remember the message. It was for me to stay strong and to never stop believing in God's love.

Another comforting moment happened when a male nurse who had been working with Ben in the ER saw I was there. Even though he wasn't officially assigned to me, he came in my room, gave me the biggest bear hug, and told me to just hang on. He knew the severity of the situation, and even though these medical professionals see death and injury every day, he took the time to come in and tell me he cared. They found no injuries aside from a hematoma on my thigh where my seatbelt had been holding my body when the car flipped. They gave me some anxiety medicine and some painkillers for my leg, and I practically ran back upstairs.

As the morning progressed, more friends from Statesboro arrived at the hospital. My parents were en route from Illinois, catching a flight from St. Louis. David was awake, and since I had not slept at all yet, told me I needed to try to get some sleep. Someone from the hospital found an empty room upstairs in the Children's Hospital, and I was sent up there. I took the pills and fell into a restless sleep.

A couple of hours later, I woke and immediately went back down to the PICU.

Brian's situation had not changed much by this point. Ben, however, had already shown enough improvement that he was being moved to the Children's Hospital floor. While this was great news, it was still overshadowed by the seriousness of Brian's situation. Before Ben was taken upstairs, we brought him in to see his brother. In my mind, I truly thought this might be the last time that Ben saw Brian alive. Brian bore little resemblance to himself, lying there comatose. How we explained the situation to Ben, I can't remember. We just prayed together, and the four of us were reunited in Brian's room for that short while.

Eventually, Ben did have to be sent upstairs, and thankfully, our amazing friends took over being Ben's primary companion, guardian, and entertainment. Over the next few days, until Ben was released from the hospital, we tried to take turns spending time with him in his room, but David and I felt anxious when leaving Brian's side. We wanted to be in both places at once and couldn't. We knew Ben was going to be okay, and our friends and family would be the support he needed if we couldn't be there. A heartbreaking reality of the situation we were in was anticipating during that first weekend that any moment would be Brian's last.

3

Prayers from Around the World

My parents had flown in from Illinois, and were thankfully able to stay with a former pastor of my in-laws' church who now lived in Savannah. Their presence was comforting; they especially took over tending to Ben. One of my siblings, Dennis, lives in South Korea, and my mom had communicated to him what was going on. Naturally Dennis's family sent their love and prayers, and asked my mom to relay the message. We had no way of knowing this message would spark a prayer chain that literally spanned the world.

My mom said to Ben, "I talked to your Uncle Dennis, and he wanted me to tell you that he and Aunt Hanna are praying for you and Brian all the way in South Korea. So people are praying for you all over the world!" Ben replied (in a fashion not uncommon for him, more precocious than argumentative), "Well, technically we don't know anyone in Fiji, so we don't really have prayers from *all* over the world." We got a chuckle out of his parsing of the words, but that day, as the story was told and re-told to the friends and family waiting and praying for Brian, an idea emerged. Could they find someone who has any connection to Fiji and satisfy Ben's request?

The era of social media makes the rest of this story possible. So many friends had already been following what was going on via Facebook, and when a few key folks posted a request to try to find a person in Fiji to pray for the boys, it went viral. What began to happen completely amazed all of us. People all over the country, and then the world, began to see the posts (which were reposted dozens and dozens of times) and reply. We began to hear things like "I'm not in Fiji, but here in Germany we are praying for you" or "Prayers from Montana." The word was spreading to total strangers, friends of friends of friends, and for some reason, this prayer request compelled those who heard it not only to act with prayers of their own, but to forward it on—and on and on!

Joe began trying to track the responses of where prayers were coming from, and eventually my sister-in-law, Jennifer, brought to the waiting room a map of the world on cardboard backing. Pushpins were placed in all the locations, states, and countries we had heard people were praying. People sent word that they were on cross-country airplane flights and to know they prayed for the boys while crossing so many different states. The country list grew and grew . . . Europe, Asia, Africa, even Australia. As time went on, the group of folks waiting and praying used the word of another country as a rallying cry. People would walk in the room and simply say "Ghana!" or "Russia!" Missionaries in China, nuns in Louisiana, even staff at the Vatican, all sent in notice: they were praying for our boys. It actually didn't take long at all in the process when the word came around, "We got prayers from Fiji!"

In all honesty, Ben was somewhat unaware of this phenomenon as it was happening, or perhaps not as affected. It was a real point of hope for those of us who knew all too well the seriousness of Brian's condition, and had such heavy hearts as we waited for the seventy-two-hour window to close. Regardless, Ben did love seeing the map, which we proudly brought up to his room with pushpins covering it! The United States was completely covered, in fact every state eventually had at least one (most had many) pushpins. Europe, as well, had nearly every country. Even places you would never expect, like The Congo, India, Afghanistan, and New Zealand. It became Joe's mission to not stop there. Since every continent except for Antarctica was covered with pins, Joe decided to use the Internet to find a researcher or scientist working there to add to our prayer chain. After a search engine provided some contacts, he e-mailed these total strangers out of the blue, explained the story, and sure enough, got a response almost immediately. Even in Antarctica, in the furthest reaches of this planet, people prayed.

Another amazing example of the power of this story occurred when Joe's friend from Wisconsin happened to see his post. By now a picture of the prayer map was appearing on many of our friends' Facebook pages, and the sight of it kept inspiring more and more locations to be sent to us. Joe's friend worked for Lands' End (the clothing retailer) and offered to share the picture and the story (minus specifics of our location and last name for privacy) on their Lands' End Facebook page. At that time of year in particular, with so many people Christmas shopping, their site received many hits each day. We agreed, and Lands' End shared the story, asking their customers to add a "virtual pushpin" for our boys. Over twenty-seven hundred total strangers added their prayers and good wishes via this page, so much that we did finally give up on trying to place pins for every response received.

Lands' End didn't stop there though. The company put together a package of goodies to be sent to the boys, and hoped it would be possible to find a local person to dress as Santa to deliver the presents, and then add a pushpin for the North Pole. The hospital minister gladly obliged to play Santa, and a great, happy memory of this time was seeing him come in Ben's room with a bag full of gifts. Ben, being ten years old, played along and was most surprised when "Santa" said he had brought two visitors in on the sleigh as well. My brother Tim and sister Bridget, having just arrived from Illinois that day, got to be a part of the surprise in that way. In the end, the company went above and beyond to try to help our family in this terrible time.

So why did this happen? Was it because it was the Christmas season? Was it because of Ben's quick wit that people just enjoyed? Was it because of the heartbreaking idea of a boy recovering from his own serious injuries all while fearing that he may lose his little brother? Something about this story hit a nerve. I ponder what it was that caused the tidal wave of prayers to spread and spread, and am still in awe to this day when I look at that map to see that the world was united in prayers for my family. There are many poignant and amazing pieces to this story, but the evidence of people's goodness and faith in God that this prayer map evoked may be one of the most touching.

In our darkest hour, when David and I could barely hold on to make it through the day, the *world* had our backs. The prayers of strangers hit heaven like a prayer tsunami, waves and waves of prayer crashing upward. To this day, we still continue to hear that people who began to pray for Brian and Ben that weekend keep us in their daily prayers. Their *daily* prayers! I am so humbled by this, and so aware that in that moment, God provided for us this community (of both friends and strangers) to do the heavy lifting. How many people connected to God in those moments? How many said a prayer for the first time in perhaps months or years? I see this phenomenon as one of the most beautiful things that could have come from a tragedy like a seven-year-old boy on his deathbed from a brain injury.

4

The Waiting Game

The seventy-two-hour window came to an end. The doctors were still pessimistic about Brian's prognosis. A neurological test was ordered, which in effect would determine if Brian was actually in their terms "brain dead," and honestly, all indications pointed to this conclusion. As a parent, it's still impossible to describe the feeling of that morning, thinking that a terrible situation is about to get even worse.

The neurologist began the exam. They poked and prodded Brian, looking for reflex reactions, but also intentional ones. During a portion of the exam, Brian moved his limbs away from the place they were pinching him. Intentional movement to escape the discomfort of them pinching him! This was not what the doctor expected to happen. The horrible prognosis that he was already gone was wrong. The look of surprise on the neurologist's face said it all . . . despite every medical reason why he shouldn't, Brian survived this critical time. David and I had asked for Father Brett Brannen to be there with us. He was the priest from our former parish in Statesboro whom we had briefly met earlier that fall, as he had arrived to town around the same time we had moved. Even though the physical examination seemed surprising and positive, I still didn't know what the doctors were thinking. All of us were ushered to a separate room and shown a CT scan of Brian's brain. I just kept trying to figure out what was happening. Finally, it was Father Brett that asked the doctor, "Are you saying you no longer think Brian's injury is life-threatening at this time?" and the doctor said he believed Brian was not in immediate danger of dying and was definitely not brain-dead.

Hearing this was like being released from a prison of fear and anxiety. I am sure the medical staff still had plenty of negative things to say, but in effect, they said that Brian's brain shouldn't be swelling any further at this point, and that he was likely spared from the fatal brain stem compression they expected initially. We went out to the waiting room filled with people to announce the good news. "Good" was relative at that time, but this was the first non-catastrophic piece of information we'd been given about Brian in three days, and we rejoiced over it and thanked God for bringing him through that terrible time.

Later during Brian's stay, someone slipped me a handwritten letter from a medical student who had been part of the team following the neurosurgeon around on that rotation.

Then there was the miracle on Tuesday morning when Brian moved. Let no one tell you otherwise . . . we witnessed a miracle this week. It was a wonderful feeling to be dead wrong about what medicine seemed to indicate. It was a humbling reminder of who is ultimately in control. It is a lesson I plan to hold closely with me as I move forward in my career as a physician.

He closed his letter with Romans 8:18: "I consider that our present sufferings are not worth comparing with the glory that will one day be revealed in us," to which he added, "including Brian." To this day, I carry this note in my wallet and read it from time to time. It reminds me that God is always working in the worst of situations and causing good to happen in the world. How many patients in the future will that doctor ultimately treat, and how will seeing the power of prayer and faith change how he deals with the lives of those he is working to help? It's a beautiful reminder to always look for the good.

5

Memorial: Part One

A social worker had suggested during one of our first days in the hospital that we should try to get a room at the Ronald McDonald House (RMH), located right across the parking lot from the hospital. At first, we were told they were full, but the director decided to let us stay for one night in the weekend manager's room (which was open at that time). David set up the arrangements, but late one evening I needed to go over and check-in myself. I sat across the desk from the kind staff member in total disbelief that I was there. She was so reassuring and positive and told me, "We've seen so many miracles here." I remember thinking, *I may not even be here another night . . . a miracle is so far beyond my comprehension.* But as it turns out, she was right! As the days went by, we were eventually given a regular room with a private bath, and began to settle in to our routine of waking up at the RMH and heading straight over to Brian's room. Food was there for the taking (not that I wanted to eat anything), but the coffee was a blessing on those early mornings.

Every bedroom at the RMH had a white board on the door, many of which had encouraging notes or messages displayed. One day during our first week, I wrote part of the lyrics to a song that had been running through my mind at that time on our board. A Tom Petty rock anthem might be a surprising place to find comfort, but one in particular seemed so appropriate for what we were feeling at that point. Every time I came back to our room and saw that phrase, "We won't back down," it felt empowering and encouraging.

Four days after the accident, Ben was released from the hospital, and was moved to his grandparents' house in Statesboro, where his grandma and aunt cared for him. Around that same time, my father-in-law was released to go home as well. Having Ben an hour away was very tough, and yet, we knew being in the comfortable surroundings of his grandparents' place was the best option. Many friends and classmates of his began to visit him and keep him as entertained as possible. It was already determined he would not be cleared to return to school until after the winter break in January, so all he really needed to do was recuperate. He was scheduled to begin some physical therapy, as he had trouble walking at first due to a pelvic fracture, and he came to Savannah for that therapy, giving us a chance to see him when he was there. A week or so after being released, he was caught doing wheelies and tricks on his walker, at which point everyone agreed, he was definitely getting better and we could get rid of the walker!

Brian's condition during the first week after the accident could be described as serious and still critical due to his brain injury. Amazingly, he had not sustained any significant injuries to his body; no internal injuries, no skin lacerations, no broken bones except for a hairline pelvic bone fracture. Concerns were very high surrounding his eyes; without the ability to keep his eyes open, the corneas were becoming scratched. He risked getting an infection that could have taken his sight, and treatment for this issue began. The pressure monitor in his head stayed in, and the levels just stayed high. Any small decrease or change we celebrated; however, we could see the medical staff never showed much optimism.

The nursing staff at the PICU will forever have my gratitude and love, however, because many of them made getting through the days there possible for us. After brief and pessimistic doctor visits each morning, the nurses would explain details further and answer our questions more compassionately and with such kindness. They treated Brian with such gentleness and love and wanted to hear about him—what kind of kid was he, what did he like to do, what motivated him. In a clinical medical setting, patients often just become another case, a number. Not all of the doctors made us feel this way, but I can say that *none* of the nurses did.

David and I valued those nurses even more as day by day we sat by Brian's bedside praying everything would be okay somehow. Some days were spiked with elements of hope, others felt just like the world was ending no matter what we tried to believe. He remained unconscious and unresponsive, partially because of medication being given to him to relieve his brain from processing (and therefore give it the ability to heal) and partially because of the extent of his injury. The side of his head where the skull piece had been removed was grotesquely swollen, and raised inches above where his skull would have been. Because of this precarious condition, he couldn't be moved easily, and we really couldn't hold him or get in the bed with him. We had to simply hold his hand and touch and stroke his chest and cheeks while we sat by his bed and talked, sang, and prayed over him.

Given the prognosis following that seventy-two-hour window seemed to indicate that further improvement would come, the family and friends who had been present went back home to their families. We were introduced to a way in which we could keep all these friends at a distance updated on Brian's progress, a non-profit called CaringBridge, which allows families to set up a website/blog that others could subscribe to in order to receive updates. What a blessing that became to David and me! As it was so difficult to talk about some of the things happening, and would have been very time consuming to actually speak with everyone, we relied on our blog to keep the many friends and family updated. As the Facebook messages had resonated, so too did the CaringBridge blog. Many friends shared and shared, and we continued to have people joining the site in order to follow Brian's progress. In addition, two separate groups were created on Facebook for those

"Praying for the Murkison Family." We did our best to update both places; however, the CaringBridge was our preferred method of writing and reflecting.

It was almost eerie how much comfort and strength seemed to come after each post went out to those reading. We heard from so many people in the message board giving us words of encouragement and love, I have to admit it was almost addictive to write something. Shortly after we did, a boomerang of love and compassion just came back to us and lifted us up. In particular, Brian's first grade teacher, Terri Williams, wrote to us the week after the accident and sent us a beautiful message:

 When we were talking, I asked the kids to talk about some things they like about Brian. I jotted down some of these comments. Here they are:

* He is on the highest level in the class on "Math Facts in a Flash."
* He makes us have running races on the playground and he always wins.
* He sits next to me and tells me the words when we are reading aloud.
* He is funny and makes me laugh.
* He is my best friend.
* He never has to sign the "Behavior Log."
* He is good on the computer.
* He always finishes his work on time.
* He is nice to everyone.

For us at that time, every shred of normalcy was cherished. We appreciated so much being able to laugh and smile at the kids' comments. We found inspiration and humor in hearing about Brian instigating races only so he could win, and we thought about that competitive spirit and how it was helping him in his recovery. We saw some signs of him being "in there" fighting to get better. Some days when the nurses had to change his tubes or IVs, he would bat his arm up to push them away. Other times when they suctioned out his lungs (to remove mucous that develops from being bedridden), he would squirm and struggle as anyone would if a suction tube was being sent down your throat. But throughout these two weeks, the doctors' prognosis only remained bleak. At one point, we were given the prediction that any recovery he might have would take months if not years. In our world of relatively immediate response, even in medical settings, hearing that the path forward was uncertain and rocky, and the only thing they could really predict would be that it would take a long time, was so difficult. Compared to Ben's injuries, which were acute, we began to receive information about what Traumatic Brain Injury (TBI) really means—a chronic, life-long impairment. It was only our community of supporters who helped us keep it together during that time.

6

The Darkest Hour

As the second week came to a close, the sedative medications were finally drawn down to a low enough level that the doctors felt a true assessment could be made of Brian's current brain function. The metal pressure monitor in his head had prevented them from being able to conduct an MRI scan up until that point. However, it was finally decided the monitor would come out, and the MRI was scheduled for Friday morning, two weeks since the day of the accident.

A nervous knot tied my stomach up that morning. I remember sitting in Brian's room waiting for him to return from the MRI and the nurse making me eat something. I think she knew I needed my strength for what came next. We knew once the test was completed the doctors were going to conference and discuss what the results meant, and would be sitting down with David and me to tell us their prognosis at that point. We had seen enough negative feedback from the doctors already that we knew we might get a serious and potentially catastrophic answer. We asked Joe and Kristen and our new friend Rachel (one of the hospital chaplains) to be with us as we received the news.

The room they chose for us to meet in was tiny, a private waiting room probably meant for four or maybe five people. I cannot remember how many of us there were, but I do remember that several folks had to stand or sit on the floor. The neurosurgeon was the team leader, and was the one to speak. He told us the damage that could be seen by the MRI (and that the CT scans were not able to assess) was beyond something that could be overcome. The entire team had reviewed the scans and concurred. Damage to parts of Brian's brain stem and middle brain were significant. In addition, the swelling of the brain had still not relapsed as usually occurs in a recovery.

We were told in very specific detail that we had the option to continue to pursue treatment, but the best prediction the team had was if Brian were to survive, there would be no foreseeable time in the future that he would ever awaken. He would never eat, drink, or speak again. He would never have control of his body, and would be completely bedridden. He would have no way to communicate, nor would he likely have any way of even knowing who or where he was, or be cognizant of anything. The normally aloof and blunt neurosurgeon was in tears as he explained this to us, and answered David's question of "Have you ever seen anyone recover from an injury this severe?" with a sorrowful "No." He told us if this was his own young son, he would not pursue further medical intervention, so strong was his certainty that this was irreparable damage.

The doctors left. We sat in stunned silence with Joe, Kristen, and Rachel. At some point, we all just ended up sitting together in a circle and praying. What we prayed for, I don't remember, and I think God's mercy gives us a form of amnesia when it comes to certain memories that are just too difficult to come back. We eventually left the hospital, and Joe and Kristen drove us out to the beach at Tybee Island. It was a sunny day. David and I walked onto the sand, having barely been able to speak following the conference. We sat down, held on to each other, and prayed we would know the right thing to do.

With all my heart, I believed that heaven (or the afterlife, or whatever you want to call it) was a real and true state. I believed too that God loved Brian, and although it was difficult to believe it was possible that anyone (even God) could love Brian more than we did, I knew it was true. To imagine Brian suffering a life of being a vegetable, not having any chance of anything like the life he had lived, was unbearable. It wasn't a moment of giving up so much as a surrendering to God what was God's. He gave us the beautiful gift of our son, and it seemed in that moment, he was asking us to offer him back. The image of Brian in heaven being free of pain and worry, laughing, playing, being with God for eternity was clear in my head. It made the decision we had to make possible.

We returned to the hospital. We sought a second opinion, and the same answer came back. There was no hope of meaningful recovery. Later that day, we made our wishes known to the medical team. The next morning they would remove Brian's ventilator and discontinue extraordinary means of medical support. We made a critical decision at that time to not remove Brian's ng-tube—his source of water and nutrition—though some on the team encouraged us to do this, unbelievably to me, to "speed things up." He would remain on pain medications, and we were told once the ventilator was removed, he would fail to bring in enough oxygen and quietly pass. It was said that it could be a matter of minutes or hours, they could not be certain, but that this would be the way in which Brian's heart would eventually stop beating.

We made no mention on our CaringBridge page of this devastating news, but spoke with our parents and told them of our decision. The next morning, Ben was brought back to Savannah, and we prepared him the best we could for the news that Brian was not going to make it. How heartbreaking it still is to picture our still-injured Ben being as strong as he could be, yet facing the worst possible news of his life, that he was about to lose his brother. A child-life specialist from the hospital came in and helped Ben make a handprint of both he and Brian, which they would frame for us as a keepsake. They also cast Brian's hand in plaster, so we could keep a reminder of his physical body with us after he was gone. All in all, the morning was incredibly difficult and yet moving and filled with love. Ben asked if there was any way the doctors could be wrong, and we were so sad to tell him we didn't think they were.

I could not force myself to be in the room when the ventilator came out. Prior to this day, we had seen Brian breathing on his own in addition to the breaths being provided by the ventilator, so we knew he had the capacity (though limited) for breathing, and therefore didn't expect him to stop breathing immediately. Without the intrusion of the breathing tube and the pressure monitor on his head, we were able to dress Brian in some of his clothes, instead of the hospital gown. The time had passed for caution regarding causing further damage to him by being in the bed with him, so I climbed in, and for the first time in two weeks, cradled and held my baby in my arms. We prayed for peace for him and for us. I felt at the time that in choosing this for Brian, it relieved him of the suffering, and I would take it on myself . . . *for* him.

Through God's grace, David and I tried to fill the space with light and love. We sang and talked to Brian, and the hours passed. The nurses monitored his oxygen level, and at one point, we saw it dipping, so much that they discouraged us from even leaving to use the bathroom, thinking the end was imminent. However, the day turned into night. We would check with the nurse before even contemplating setting a foot outside his room, but at one point they said, he's stabilized at the moment, and one of us at a time could step out, but only for the briefest of minutes. We stayed in his room all night, watching some of his favorite TV shows and hoping he would somehow hear the audio. The next morning, we eventually put the message out on our CaringBridge site that Brian's death was imminent. I can see how it shocked and confused people, because though we had tried to convey the gravity of his case, I think most wanted to believe that any child can recover from an injury. We had shared some positive turns, and that had given people reason to believe the positive would outweigh the negative. Prayers continued to pour in, and we asked everyone to please just pray for peace for him and for us.

Another night came, and yet, he was somehow still with us. I imagined God being gentle with us as if he was saying, "You have chosen the right thing, now I am giving you this precious time to say good-bye to your Brian." I think we must have told Brian how much we loved him one million times over that weekend. But I very clearly remember also telling him, "I love you with all my heart, Brian, and I can't even understand how, but Jesus loves you even more than me. He wants you to come be with him." Through it all, Brian's eyes never opened, he just kept breathing, he just kept living.

Monday morning came. Some on the medical staff again proposed we remove his food and water supply, to bring closure. We refused. We were then advised (kindly) that the PICU was not really set up for palliative care, and they would like us to consider moving Brian. They offered an unused and quieter room of the PICU, but felt that bringing him home with a hospice nurse would be a better option. We could not have returned to our home in Atlanta 250 miles away from our support network, but called and found out a bed was available at the Ogeechee Area Hospice in Statesboro. We made the arrangements to move him and waited for the ambulance. I will never forget one of the nurses who had been so caring and loving to us was on duty that morning, and so desperately wanted to travel with Brian in the ambulance. Unfortunately, it was the holiday season, and there were no extra nurses on duty that day, so she had to remain. The tears in her eyes and the hug she gave me were so sincere. I knew she hated saying good-bye to us.

David rode in the ambulance, and I (somehow) drove our car the fifty miles back to Statesboro. We were welcomed into a building filled with peace and love by staff members and nurses who made us feel immediately comforted. As terrible as the past two weeks had been, being in the calm environment there took some anxiety away from our hearts. My reflection that day on CaringBridge says it best:

Tonight, Brian lies peacefully in his beautiful room here at the hospice. He is breathing on his own. He is calm. He looks like he is asleep. And now David and I can begin to let down our guard a little and let the people we love most surround us and hold us up, in the place Brian knew as home for most of his life, and the place we love so much. Ben is less than ten minutes away, and we are thrilled that we no longer have to go days without seeing him. We must face what still lies ahead, but we have the community here in person (and here on this site from everywhere) to make it.

7

Asking for a Miracle

Alone behind the wheel, I slowly turned right onto a small, narrow, gravelly road—the kind I used to drive by on my way to the mall, or a soccer game, or a friend's house. The single lane at the Eastside Cemetery, Statesboro, Georgia, made a path amidst the tombstones to my left and my right. Sometimes I used to see a tent erected over the plot or even see the parked cars of the family and friends standing at the grave for a service. And I kept on driving, turned up the radio, looked away, distracted myself from thinking about it, or at most said a quick prayer for whomever that might be back there.

In my youth, going to the cemetery was a fairly normal thing. My family had dealt with death plenty by the time I was Ben's age. My paternal grandfather, a grandmother-like great aunt, even my own little brother passed from a crib death when I was only seven. Add countless more cousins, family friends, or relatives that passed during my formative years, and going to a funeral home or cemetery was just not that big a deal. We said the rosary at the visitation. We went to the funeral mass and graveside service. Every Memorial Day my dad would gather huge arms-full of peonies that grew in our yard and bring them to decorate his parents' grave. Right next to grandpa and grandma, my brother Peter (only fourteen months old when he died). We would kneel, pray, and leave our flowers. The cemetery—I knew it well.

My own children had never really experienced any of the above, at least not due to an actual death. Ironically, in November one week before the accident while visiting my parents, we took the boys for the first time to a cemetery in Keokuk, Iowa, to see the grave of my maternal grandparents. It was not uncomfortable for them so much as interesting. As in a "hmm, we've never done *this* before on one of our trips" kind of way. Ben in particular was much more interested in the National Cemetery that was adjacent, finding gravestones of fallen military members from all of the branches, and going back to the late 1800s. For a kid interested in military history, this was a little more compelling. But the whole rest of it, not so much.

Odd, too, that just a few weeks prior to that, Ben and I had been out taking a walk for exercise and the subject of heaven came up. Not that we've never talked about it in general terms, obviously Ben knew what heaven was, but this conversation was different. We began to talk about the fact that sooner or later someone that Ben knew well was going to die. At the time I really didn't know what possessed me to want to impress this upon him, but I really felt compelled to talk about what happens to someone once they pass away. Ben was his typical good sport about the whole thing, making jokes and saying that he imagined that heaven would be a scene like this: "You're in heaven and you're like, 'Hey, I would really love a candy bar' and then you reach into your pocket, and *there's a candy bar!*" We laughed, and yet, I was relieved that we'd had the discussion. I recalled this conversation when driving through the cemetery while Brian lay in a hospice across town and knew in my heart that God had led me to have this talk with Ben on that day. It was one of many "coincidences" that I believed were nothing of the kind; they were messages that God was sending to help us for what was to come.

My head was full of questions as I drove slowly through the plots. Why did I come here alone? Why haven't I been able to talk to David about this yet? How will we know what to do, how to have a funeral? We had faced so much already, and we knew the details of Brian's death would have to be dealt with, yet we couldn't bring ourselves to discuss anything other than to agree we would bury him in Statesboro. The part of me that must be a planner had brought me to this place, if nothing else to visualize where it was going to be that our sweet boy would be laid to rest. I hated the thought that I may someday regret making a hasty or wrong decision about the details. As bizarre as it sounds even to me, it was a mechanism to not think about the big picture of what his death would mean. It was a distraction (albeit morbid) of "What casket would we choose?" and "Are there any nice plots left that aren't by the road?" I finally realized I was gaining nothing from my time in the cemetery, and headed back to the hospice on that gray December day. I felt as confused and hopeless as I had before.

Psychologically it became very difficult to deal with the fact that we were going to lose him, yet he was not yet gone. We were in a type of purgatory, he wasn't gone and he wasn't with us either. During this time, the magnitude of the prayers for him and us ramped up.

The fourth night after he was removed from the ventilator, two prayer vigils occurred. One in Atlanta, the other in Statesboro. All over the country, those who couldn't attend either vigil in person lit candles in their homes and prayed for our family. The power of these prayers was real. We did not know at the time if Brian would even make it through another night, and yet, we felt buoyed by the intentions of others and asked for prayers of peace and for our family to recover from this loss.

What I did not expect is that God wanted more from me. When the sixth night came and Brian was still breathing, Ben expressed to us that he really didn't believe Brian was going to die, and that he wanted to pray for a Christmas miracle. It became clear to me what God really wanted. I imagine it as if I had been on the edge of a cliff. I had stood on that edge and asked for God to give me the strength to hold on, but I finally realized he didn't want me to hold on, he wanted me to jump. He wanted me to surrender it all and trust that he was in control. To give over my rational, human-oriented thoughts that told me there was no way Brian could recover and to ask God for a supernatural experience, for a miracle. That night as David and I both wrote on our blog asking for everyone following our story to stop praying for peace in Brian's passing but to instead shift the intention to an actual miracle, I jumped off that cliff. And in God's beautiful love for me, he not only caught me, he lifted me up higher than I could have imagined. I know now that God wanted me to put *all* my faith in him. To risk that we would feel worse if we prayed for a miracle and Brian died anyway. It took all the courage I had, but I decided to ask for the miracle we needed.

 All of the love, faith, devotion, and care shown by you is already a miracle. God, please, continue to bless this child with miracles, and bring him back to health so he may live on, and this will spread your love even more. David and I prayed tonight that Mother Mary and Joseph would intercede for Brian that St. George, the patron saint of scouts, would intercede for Brian. We pray that the Lord Jesus hears all of your prayers and that we continue to believe that through him, nothing is impossible.

That night Brian began to heal. By the following morning, we were observing a radically different child.

 We can feel your prayers for a miracle, the light and the air and energy in this room have changed. Brian's color is better, his lungs are clear, and the swelling in his head has gone down *significantly* since yesterday. We are putting 1000% energy toward prayer for this recovery now. We see this boy fighting with everything in him, defying all odds.

Trust in God. Faith in God. Never have these words rang more true than seeing the physical changes apparent in Brian that morning. My prayer had been answered, and then some. Because we had put ourselves out there for the world to see, our miracle was not just "ours." It belonged to every person praying for our family. It changed hearts and minds; it brought people closer to God. I *finally* knew in my heart that Brian would fully recover, and I began to pray for his *complete* recovery from these injuries. I gave God my promise that I would do whatever it took—no matter how many hours of rehabilitation, no matter what doctors we had to find, anything he needed of me—if he would bring our Brian back.

My belief that he was doing just that has literally been my motivation and strength ever since. In times of struggle and pain during the process, I could cling to my firm belief that this was part of the deal. God had not taken him, and therefore, I had faith it was because Brian could be, and *would be*, fully healed one day. How beautiful it is now to be able to look back on that leap of faith and know how right it was to trust in God's power. I am so grateful that I jumped.

8

Christmas at a Hospice

During the week at hospice, Brian received some of the kindest, most loving care he could have ever experienced, and we will always be grateful to the nurses and staff there. David and I had so many people offering us cards, books, food, gift certificates to restaurants, prayers, and even religious articles. Being only three miles away from Ben instead of nearly sixty was a huge comfort to us as well. We slept in Brian's hospice room, alternating a cushioned window seat/futon and a recliner. Though I am sure our friends and family made us eat, I don't remember ever wanting to. We were in survival mode, and spent many hours listening to soft Christmas music and praying. It was the week of Christmas, a time we expected to be on a family ski trip then home preparing just like any other family would for the biggest holiday of the year. Instead, we found ourselves living this bizarre existence.

Because we felt the energy shifting in Brian, David and I felt confident enough that we could both go together to Christmas Eve Mass at St. Matthews with Ben. Until that time, one of us was physically with Brian at every moment. Our mothers came together to sit with Brian while we went to the Mass. I remember watching Ben help carry in the statue of the baby Jesus to the manger on the altar during the procession. I remember hearing the music and feeling the joy and love in that church on one of the holiest nights of the year. And even though on the surface you would think any mother whose seven-year-old boy was a mile away in a hospice bed would be devastated, instead that night, I felt a sense of peace and hope. I wasn't crying or despairing. God had already given me the answer I needed, and so, I celebrated with my family and community in that church. My dear friend Chris, whose own children were close to Ben and Brian and who had supported us in so many ways already by that time, saw me after Mass. She asked me how Brian was and I can remember saying, "He had a really good day today," with a smile on my face.

For all of my thirty-nine years at that time, I don't ever remember having a "bad" Christmas. Until I was out of college, I spent the holiday at home with my parents and siblings. After David and I got married, we alternated whose family we would share Christmas with, and we were so blessed to be part of two great families, so it was always fun and festive. After Ben was born, we celebrated in an even more poignant way, enjoying showering our eight-month-old baby with far too many gifts on his first Christmas, and loving the chance to re-live the magic of that time of year that is somewhat diminished when you're spending it with only adults. By the time Ben was about two, we made the decision that we would always wake up in our own home on Christmas morning. I just always wanted my kids to have the memories like I did of arriving at the tree pajama-clad, finding what Santa had left, and then getting to spend the rest of the day at home enjoying those gifts. My parents, who were so far away from Georgia, were especially gracious about the change, since unlike my in-laws who lived close enough to come for the day to our house, they would be missing having us with them. I remember my mom saying something like, "I got to have all of you kids here at home for twenty-five Christmases, it's alright that you want to do the same for your kids." Brian's first Christmas came when he was only nine weeks old. Such an adorable, little, chubby infant, I was excited to buy matching PJs for him and Ben. We have precious pictures of three-year-old Ben holding his little brother on the sofa, both in identical green Christmas pajamas.

That year we had it all planned. (As a person who really loves to plan, I kind of always hated the expression "we plan, God laughs," but it seems like a pretty applicable point now.) We would go on a ski trip to North Carolina then come home to Atlanta to host Christmas for David's family. I would cook, haul out the mostly unused china and fancy stemware, and the boys would enjoy their presents all day. We thought we would go out to a local park called Stone Mountain that hosts a Christmas festival. I definitely thought on December 1 of that year that I would have been able to predict with 95 percent accuracy how that day would be.

Instead, I woke up Christmas morning in a hospice to the sight of my precious seven-year-old son still lying comatose. How amazing would it have been if instead of that we had awoken to see Brian awake and talking to us (the way Ben was imagining what a Christmas miracle looks like)? That, however, was not what I saw. My heart and mind had been changed though, and it was as if I was able to react to those realities with an understanding that wasn't completely rational, yet which has proven to be 100 percent correct! It was awful and sad to be in a hospice on that morning instead of watching my kids opening their gifts. But it was not primarily a feeling a grief I felt that morning, but instead one of peace. Someone shared with us on our CaringBridge around this time that we were not *waiting for* a miracle; we were in the process of the miracle unfolding already. When I read that, I felt immediately that it was spot-on right. The miracle had already begun to unfold, who said it needed to look like some Hollywood soap opera version when someone in a coma is suddenly perfectly fine?

Over at my in-laws' house, Christmas morning was going to happen much like we had anticipated it would have at our house. David's brother Jimmy, his wife Elisabeth, and their daughters had flown in from Seattle once we shared the news that Brian would not make it. They did manage to arrive in time to come and visit him while he was still in the hospital, and definitely were there at some point each day of our time at the hospice. As they lived so far away, it was a special holiday for the grandparents to get to have their granddaughters with them on Christmas morning, especially Lucy who was having her first Christmas. Ben, who was still living there along with Jennifer, my sister-in-law, rounded out the group.

Newly confident that Brian was on a path to recovery, David and I took turns driving over to the house that morning to spend a little "normal" time. After all the other presents had been opened, there was one left with no name on it. Among other things, Ben had asked for a cell phone for Christmas. The world is certainly a different one now because it's not that strange for a fifth grader to have a phone, but that year, buying it was only a desire on David and my part to do whatever we could for Ben, even getting him something we had previously said he really didn't need. Jennifer and I arranged that she would leave the room and call Ben's new cell number. Ben's surprise and happiness when he was encouraged to find out why that box is ringing was a great memory. But just a few minutes later, watching him and his little cousins playing underneath the tree, I became overwhelmed by my emotions. It wasn't right. Brian should have been there. I couldn't stay and be there knowing how unfair it was that Brian was missing this. As I arrived back at the hospice, it was actually easier for me, as odd as that is. There I could focus on praying for Brian, and tried to fill his room up with as much love and happiness as I could.

We had many family and friends come by on that rainy Christmas to visit Brian and us. Many had seen him a few days before, and were astonished by his physical changes. Our new spiritual mentor Fr. Brett, the priest from Statesboro who had been down to Savannah to help us so many times, came by late that afternoon, and we shared with him our belief that a miracle really was what God wanted us to ask for. He told us that he has seen real physical miracles before, and though we can never know what God plans, it wasn't wrong to ask for this. He said we could look at it this way. What was going against a miracle for Brian was a devastating brain injury. What was going for a miracle were thousands of prayers being sent up on his behalf, excellent medical care, and most importantly, a seven-year-old with an amazing spirit and an otherwise healthy body who had already shown the ability to do something no one thought possible. As David wrote on our journal that night, when you look at it that way, we liked our chances.

9

Transitioning

During his time at hospice, Brian received nutrition and water and pain medication, but no other real medical interventions, though our former family practitioner Dr. Carla Branch did come to check on Brian each day. She, like the doctors in Savannah, expected that eventually Brian's lungs would fail to provide enough oxygen to his brain, and he would very peacefully pass. However, as time went on, she began to share that he was not showing the signs of someone who was beginning the process of dying. As a physician, she was keenly aware of physical clues that begin to appear when the end is near. Because of the holiday, she did not plan to see Brian on Christmas Day, but did pay a visit the following day. We had begun to see the physical changes I have already described, and though fearful of the answer, we talked with her about having another neurological test performed on Brian. She agreed it was time, because it made no sense not to when he was still with us more than a week after being removed from the ventilator.

On Tuesday, December 27, a neurologist from Statesboro was scheduled to come and conduct the assessment. As had been the case in the PICU, when patients are on too much pain medication, they may not be able to really show accurate response to the neurological tests. Therefore, Dr. Branch had the nurses begin to wean down the amount of pain medication Brian was receiving the evening before the test. In an effort to relieve the stress and anxiety of what that test may say, I invited our friend Kristen to come have dinner at Brian's room that Monday night.

Kristen stopped by one of my favorite restaurants in town and brought take-out Thai food, something that Brian had actually loved (surprisingly). It was a sign of my renewed faith and hope that I could let my guard down enough to enjoy a meal, and spend time laughing with our friend. I remember thinking that despite how serious the situation still was how it must be nice for Brian to have the sound of laughter in his room instead of crying or hushed speaking.

What I didn't expect was that Brian could not only hear us, but apparently could smell the delicious Thai food aroma as well. After we had been sitting bunched up at a small, rolling table in the corner of the room eating for a while, I went over to Brian's bed. I said something to him like, "I'm sorry, Brian, we were just over there eating up that yummy Thai food . . . I didn't mean to ignore you so long." Suddenly, Brian made a clear sound, as if in response to my statement! In the three weeks since the accident, he had been silent, comatose. Due to the combination of having lowered levels of sedating pain medications, hearing happy sounds, and smelling familiar scents, Brian began his return to consciousness. Kristen later wrote me she had never been quite so moved as she was seeing that sight. By the next morning, as daylight came around, Brian was consistently opening his eyes again of his own free will.

Thanks to the generosity of friends, my brother Dennis had been able to get a ticket to fly in from South Korea, and by coincidence, arrived that morning. When he walked in the room with my parents, Brian shifted his gaze to look towards the door. We were almost giddy with excitement to see those beautiful eyes open again, though he still closed them often and was clearly still heavily medicated. Eventually, my mother was sitting on the opposite side of his bed from me, and she began talking to Brian. At the time, his gaze was focused on me, and almost out of instinct, I said to him, "Brian, your

Grandma is talking to you, look at Grandma," and he absolutely turned his gaze toward my mom. Later, it became more difficult for Brian to show such clear tracking of his eyes, but I know what we saw that morning. It just gave me more and more confidence that he was indeed going to be okay.

The neurologist was delayed, and was not able to come in until nearly lunchtime. Unfortunately, the withdrawal symptoms of decreasing his pain medication so quickly were beginning to affect Brian. His breathing became labored and deep, he was showing a lot of signs of distress. In that moment, we began to wonder if we had made a mistake, and if taking him off the pain medication was going to cause him to go into some kind of cardiac arrest, or seizure. Dr. Branch was called, and the nurses were instructed to give him a bit of the medicine, but still, the minutes seemed to drag on forever while we watched Brian be in terrible pain, something that mercifully we had not seen during the weeks leading up to that point. Finally, the doctor arrived, and within a few short minutes, determined that *Brian was finally showing positive responses to the neurological tests.* The doctor had the nurse pump back up the pain meds, and Brian's episode thankfully came to an end. The doctor said he wanted to consult with our neurosurgeon in Savannah, and left to make the call.

We had not spent much time considering what would happen if he did pass the test. Suddenly we realized we needed to make a decision about where we wanted Brian to be transported if he did get to leave hospice. It took no time to decide that returning to Memorial in Savannah would be the best plan. Our other option would have been the long and more risky transport back to Atlanta. Having only lived there for three months, we had no support network like we did in Savannah and Statesboro, nor did we have any experience with any of the hospitals there. Primarily for these reasons, when the doctor came back in and said the neurosurgeon agreed the Brian should go back to the hospital, we made plans right away to send him back to Savannah.

The rest of that day was a whirlwind as my father-in-law came with boxes so that all the many gifts, cards, posters, and food that had filled the hospice room could be packed up. The ambulance was arranged, and one week and a day after we'd made the trip to hospice, Brian returned for the second time to the Pediatric ICU at Memorial in Savannah.

10

Memorial: Part Two

There are amazing people who work in pediatric intensive care units. To go to work day in and day out, knowing that every single patient in your care is in such serious condition that he or she needs to be in an ICU environment must take incredible dedication. We had come to know and respect so many of the staff at the PICU in Savannah during the two weeks we had spent there, and we knew that many of them mourned our loss when we left for hospice with Brian. I can imagine in their careers, it's not totally unusual to have some children who are "repeat" customers so to speak. But I am confident that they had never been given the chance to work with a patient who, the last they saw him, was being removed from life support and sent to hospice care. Not in a peds unit. Who has ever heard of anyone getting kicked out of hospice?

A completely huge smile was on my face as I walked next to Brian's gurney as the ambulance crew wheeled him up from the first floor to the second. As we walked through those locked double doors, it was joy and excitement I was feeling with each and every nurse and staff member we saw. "We're *back!*" I practically yelled at

53

anyone I saw, and it was later a moment of levity when we could joke about what kind of weirdo parents would be so happy to ever have their kid admitted to a PICU.

But we *were* happy. Overjoyed actually. The fear, it was still there, but I would describe it as being like a nagging hangnail or some other small physical hurt. You might notice it, it could get your attention, but if you went back to thinking about something else, you would probably forget it was there for the most part. I can remember that one of our favorite trauma doctors came in right away to examine Brian. This doctor had been off the rotation during the crucial conference that had led us on the path we had chosen, and though he was aware of what had happened, he hadn't seen Brian immediately prior to our leaving the hospital. He did several tests to assess Brian's reflexes. Originally, the doctors' diagnosis had been that Brian's brainstem was too damaged to recover; therefore, despite having finally woken from the coma, this doctor wanted to test for reflexes, first and foremost.

During Brian's neurological testing, when the doctor pinched his skin, poked him in the eye, and looked for pupil dilation by shining lights directly in his eyes, among other procedures, Brian showed positive responses. Then the doctor asked the nurse to use a syringe to put some water into Brian's nose, to check for a gag reflex. Much to his surprise, instead of gagging and choking on the water, Brian seemingly swallowed it. The doctor made the call to the neurosurgeon, the same one who had tearfully given Brian no chance, and he later arrived and did a similar exam. Again, Brian was amazingly passing these tests. I want to be clear, if Brian had been showing this level of neurological response to these physical tests the first time around, I do not think any of the doctors would have made such a certain terminal diagnosis. As it was, back at the time of that fateful MRI, they saw "proof" from the scan, coupled with dwindling physical response on these types of exams. The combination of the two was seemingly the overwhelming evidence.

Yet, after more than a whole week of being removed from all medical intervention except food, water, and pain medication, here Brian was. Doing better than ever, showing the types of responses the doctors had hoped to see all along. His situation was still critical, no doubt, but it was within the realm of possibility for a recovery. As I tearfully spoke to the neurosurgeon, he said to me something I will never forget, "Some things medicine can't explain." For a scientist (a brain surgeon no less) to admit this must be pretty strange. But in fact, he had a child in front of him that defied medical science, and he told me he was committed to pursuing aggressive measures from that point forward to save Brian. Yet, in his assessment, we were still looking at the likelihood that Brian would be permanently impaired, probably in most physical ways (talking, walking, or eating). A best-case scenario might be he would have the capacity to someday utilize assistive technology to communicate. You know, like the quadriplegics who use a pencil in their mouth to tap a keyboard in order for the computer to talk for them. No promises of anything resembling a "normal" life for him, but at that point, we were not deterred.

The trauma doctor was able to tell us that amazingly, after three weeks of being bed-ridden (the week at hospice having had no respiratory therapy at all) Brian's lungs only had a small area of congestion. The threat of pneumonia is always present when someone is in a hospital setting for that long, but the doctor told us his lungs were strong and mostly clear. Otherwise, because Brian had not sustained any other physical injury other than a pelvic fracture from where his seat belt held him (just like Ben had), there were not many other concerns that the doctors had to worry about. Healing Brian's brain was the number one priority.

I have described that the right side of Brian's head had a piece of the skull missing. It was intentionally not replaced after his surgery that first night, in order to allow his brain room to swell. The morning of Christmas Eve when we began to sense the miracle truly was unfolding, we woke to the sight of the swelling on that side of his head markedly gone. By the time we returned to Savannah, it had actually become sunken into his head, or concave. Because there was no skull bone in that area, if he leaned one way, the tissue inside would dip down, and you could see it moving. Fortunate for us, the bone that had been removed was still at the hospital, being stored in deep freezing temperatures. Whenever possible, when patients are ready for the piece of the skull to go back in, doctors try to use the patient's own bone, to make the process easier, and so the body doesn't reject it as foreign tissue. Plans were made that Brian would be put on strong antibiotics to clear up the small chest infection, and following this, surgery would be scheduled to replace the bone.

Coming back the second time, another patient was occupying Brian's previous room. This time, Brian was placed in the same room that Ben had stayed in that very first night, room seven. We started calling it "Lucky Room Seven" and said to the nurses, "Room seven is the room our kids go when they are about to get better." I don't want to understate the concern and worry we still had, but I think that the human spirit, when faced with great adversity, gravitates toward finding the positive. We had already been through the worst situation we could have ever fathomed, and yet, here we still were.

Our minds were made up, and for me at least, I did feel that doubt was almost an insult to God. He led me to put all my faith in him. I did it, and my prayers were being answered. How terrible it would have been if I had allowed myself to sink back into despair and negative thinking. In an act of faith, I practiced being positive each day. I can see now what a benefit that was to our family as a whole that David and I both could begin to devote energy of mind, body, and spirit to Brian's recovery.

As this second stay progressed, several things began to occur. The doctors told us that a rehabilitation hospital for children in Atlanta would be the next step for Brian. Once they replaced the piece of his skull and conducted a secondary operation to insert a more permanent port into his stomach for his food and water to enter (rather than the intrusive tube still inserted in his nose), Brian could be released to Atlanta. In order to assess if he was a candidate for the rehab unit, a staff member from that hospital would be flown down to see Brian in person and speak with us. It felt very nerve wracking, almost like a recruiter from a big-time college coming to talk to our kid about whether he would get a scholarship. We felt uncertain that Brian, despite how much improvement he was showing, would be considered eligible.

Our fears were relieved when we met Laura, the first of many staff members of Children's Healthcare of Atlanta (CHOA) that would change our lives for the better. She was easy to talk with, and fairly quickly reassured us that Brian could indeed be admitted to rehabilitation. She provided us with information about the unit and answered our questions; even though at the time we didn't have any idea what we were getting ourselves into. One justification for patients to be admitted to the rehab unit, even if the patient was in as poor as shape as Brian, was for the staff there to train us as parents on how to care for Brian in our home. I really had to work hard to overcome the fear that came from imagining that what they really were saying was Brian would never progress much beyond the way we saw him at that point. We just tried to remain positive, and imagined that one day Brian would be one of the success stories featured in the promotional materials for the rehabilitation hospital. The miracle boy that gave everyone else hope.

Having approval for transport once his operations were completed, all we had to do was wait. We had gotten pretty good at the waiting game. Again, so many friends and family were able to come to Savannah and visit us. Our old stomping ground, the PICU waiting room, again became our normal place to receive our visitors. A few folks we did bring back to see Brian, and tears were in everyone's eyes when they were able to see him with his eyes finally open!

Fr. Brett was one of the visitors. The very same day he was coming for a visit, our favorite trauma doctor had an earnest conversation with us. He told us this path we were on was going to be a marathon, not a sprint. As much stress as we had been through over the past four weeks, he knew we would need to take care of ourselves if we were going to be able to continue caring for Ben and Brian. He told us that Brian had twenty-four hour care with them, and that the worst had passed. He encouraged us to take a small "vacation," although even at the time it sounded ridiculous to us, something inside knew he was right. When Fr. Brett came to visit later that day, we told him what the doctor said. He immediately offered us his family's condo out on Tybee Island if we wanted to spend a couple of nights away. His parents agreed, they would be so happy if we would go and try to take a moment to rejuvenate. Despite feeling guilty about leaving Brian's side for any amount of time, we called David's parents and arranged for them to bring Ben down to join us, and we drove the sixteen miles or so from the hospital out to the beach.

Being with Ben was so lovely. The three of us hadn't been together like that for so long, and being able to be the parent of a kid who was *not* so injured was a luxury to us at that point. We bought ourselves treats and goodies at the grocery, and settled in at the condo, enjoying views of the ocean right on our porch. For someone like me, who grew up in the Midwest, the ocean has always attracted me. Having lived for many years on the coast, this beach in particular was so familiar and comforting to me. The beauty and presence of God in our natural environment can either be overlooked or cherished, and on those days, we cherished it.

David dealt with all of this stress and worry in his own way. But the beach has always been a place of happiness, reflection, and joy for him too, so I knew it was as good for him as it was me to be able to just stare at that vast ocean and begin to try to unwind. What I did not know until later was that New Year's Eve night, something amazing happened to him. Later the next year, David shared that he had prayed that night for God to give him a sign that everything was actually going to be alright, and just as he prayed this, a shooting star streaked across the sky. It was no coincidence in my mind, just another way God was showing us to be strong and to believe in his amazing love.

Maybe this was the reason for us being there all along . . . faith, in whatever form it appears, gives us strength, helps us do what may seem impossible, and gives us comfort. Once again, right when we needed it, God provided.

11

Transition to Atlanta

As we came back and waited to hear if Brian's surgery would still be able to occur on January 2, 2012, I had a wonderful surprise visit from my oldest and best childhood friend, Becky, who flew in from Chicago for a day. Seeing her in the hospital waiting room was such a great feeling, and we just talked and talked the rest of that day. Having extra moral support was so great, and I especially appreciated having additional people to talk with because our friends who had been through the entirety of this ordeal had certainly given more than most friends ever would. I still needed to rely on them, and they gladly gave of themselves (and would continue to do so for months and months), but it was great to know I could give them a "day off" and let Becky be the one to comfort me.

As the morning came, the neurosurgeon still had Brian on the schedule for that day, but because he had just been on call over the New Year's holiday when unfortunately many traumas and accidents occur, we still weren't sure if he was up for performing the surgery. As much as we were eager for this to happen, we wanted the surgeon to be in his best form. We got the word and they took Brian into surgery that afternoon. Though we had confidence this would be successful, anytime someone in Brian's state is exposed to the risk of surgery, there are valid concerns. We waited in the hospital lobby and the nurse kept us updated each hour on how things were going. Thankfully, they eventually came out to say he had done great and would be brought back up to the PICU. Only one parent could go to the recovery area and wait with Brian until he was stable enough to be moved, and David was the one who went.

Brian's thick blond hair had been shaved off partially the night of the accident in prep for the emergency surgery. All throughout the weeks at the hospital and hospice, he had a shaved patch on the front third of his head, and the rest of the hair continued to grow longer and longer. It wasn't our main concern of course, but once we realized he would be back in surgery again, we asked if the team would just cut *all* of his hair when they prepped him, so at least it would be able to grow back evenly.

Still, it was a surprise when I saw them wheeling Brian back to the PICU with his head cleanly shaven. But what was most amazing was having that piece of his skull back in place made him look so much more like himself, not the swollen and injured appearance he had all those weeks. I cried with happiness and just couldn't stop staring and saying to people, "Look how good his head looks." The stitches were many, and he did have a small drain in the back of his head to help fluids flow out, but other than that, he was beginning to look like our Brian again. What a wonderful sight.

He recovered more the next day, and then two days after this surgery, he went back in for a second surgery to place the g-tube (Gastric tube) in his stomach. It is a laparoscopic procedure, and involves hardly any of the risk that the brain surgery did earlier, but it was still a relief to get the call that he was all done and ready to get back upstairs.

Throughout this whole week, David and I had been provided a room (again) at the Ronald McDonald house, and this time, we just treasured each and every interaction we had with other parents there, the staff, and the volunteers. It was too emotionally overwhelming the first time around to even try to talk to the other parents, since no one is there because their child is healthy and fine. But thankfully, with our new-found confidence, we were able to embrace that environment a bit more the second stay. We were comfortable there, and in a warped way, it became what we knew. The couple of days right before Brian was going to be transported to Atlanta had some real anxiety in them, despite longing to return to our home for the first time in over a month; it was difficult to leave the RMH.

But the day did finally arrive. Brian's second discharge from Memorial came on January 6, 2012. This time, I went in the ambulance, and David took the turn of driving our car. We left pretty early in the morning, a sunny and clear day. The ambulance crew was professional and polite; I sat in the back of the rig on a small seat next to Brian along with one EMT, while another one drove. The 225-mile drive took the usual three and a half hours or so, and we finally arrived at the Comprehensive Inpatient Rehabilitation Unit (CIRU) of Children's Healthcare of Atlanta.

12

Rehabilitation Begins

The nursing aid knocked on the door, then quickly came in and handed me a sheet of paper. It was a schedule for the following day, detailing which therapists would be seeing Brian and at what time. In the four weeks prior to this, our lives were a roller coaster experience. With very few exceptions, there was no telling what each day would bring, and as I have already expressed, so many of the days were not just filled with questions but with dread as well. Now, the presence of a schedule. A plan. Something to rely upon to help get through each day. For someone like me, a schedule was gold.

I was already feeling a sense of hope and positivity after arriving at CIRU. From the physical surroundings (bright, colorful, and a hospital room with a huge window and lots of natural light) to the staff themselves (friendly, upbeat, professional, and positive), you felt in that space that everyone was on board to make things better. No, more than that. They were coming from an expectation that it *would* be better. The change in expectation was striking, because it meant that despite setbacks or the limitations Brian still had, the plan was to forge ahead. No looking back, and no time for negative options.

The very first doctor that examined Brian was young and energetic. He assessed Brian, and on that day, here is what I would describe that doctor would have seen. A boy lying in the bed, eyes open but glazed and distant, with not much sign of awareness or spark. Legs that were stretched out straight. Arms that were curled up like a boxer, hands clenched into fists. An incision from the most recent head surgery on his skull, and the g-tube in his stomach still fresh. Unresponsive to requests to move. In retrospect, although we had made it so far to get to that point, he was still so very injured, so very low on the scale of coma recovery, especially compared to other patients there at the CIRU. But did the doctor begin by telling us all the worst case scenarios as we had heard before? Not at all. The doctor told Brian, "Buddy, I know your body isn't doing anything your brain is telling it to do right now, but don't worry, we're gonna fix that!"

I cannot overstate how amazing that attitude was to hear. For the first time since this crisis began, I felt we had an ally in this fight who believed a recovery *was* possible. The medical team at CHOA began to immediately make adjustments to Brian's medications in hopes of helping him "clear." Clearing is a term used with brain injuries which refers to the patient beginning to regain awareness of his or her surroundings. Once I heard this phrase, it really resonated with me. I imagined Brian's brain just being enclosed in a fog. And that this fog was a good thing for him originally, because it protected and shielded him, but as we progressed further and further along, the fog was dissipating. I used to pray that God's love and spirit would shine down into Brian's actual body, and like sunlight coming through the mist, clear his mind. It felt like such a gentle and sweet image, and I think especially at that time, anything that was not anxiety- or stress-filled was such a relief.

The three main therapies provided to Brian while he was inpatient were speech, occupational, and physical. There were also therapists on staff who provided music and recreational therapy to patients. We had access to a social worker to help us with beginning to handle the paperwork and realities of what it would mean to ultimately bring Brian home from the hospital. And we had hospital chaplains who provided us moral support and who shared countless success stories of children who had been just as impaired as Brian one day walking back in the door. At the time, although I appreciated the stories, I still had a hard time making the leap to imagining how this would happen.

A neuropsychologist did an evaluation of Brian early in the process. As he was completely unable to communicate verbally, she attempted to assess him by doing things like trying to get him to sustain his gaze in one direction or another, or to close his eyes on command, things like that. Her report ultimately showed that he was still in an extremely low level of coma recovery. This was not surprising, however as she sat and talked to David and me about her report, she also began to speak to us about things like, "Once he is back in school . . ." In order to receive special education services, students do need a complete psychological test similar to this to show eligibility and to help the schools define what services could be provided. I can remember just staring at her like she was crazy. Was she really sitting there discussing him being back in school so nonchalantly, as if it was a certainty? Now I can say, she was absolutely right. It may have been seven months before it finally happened, but Brian went back to school. Her positive attitude was just another example of the way the staff at CHOA dealt with Brian, always giving the benefit of the doubt to the prospect that he would be better.

I stayed in Brian's room during his month of hospitalization. There was a "bed" of sorts for parents that was also a window seat, and the room had a private bath, and actually was fairly spacious. On the weekends, David and I would swap, and he stayed with Brian while I spent two nights at home with Ben. Ben had returned to school at this point, it was early January and the second part of the school year had begun. The school was incredibly supportive, even allowing Ben to be signed up for the after-school program at the last minute so we did not have to scramble to find a place for him to go each afternoon, since I was at the hospital, and David usually didn't return home until about six p.m. He was happy to be back in a routine, and ultimately did pretty well during that month, despite our lives having changed so dramatically.

Our neighbors in Atlanta provided us snacks and dinners each week, and several came to the hospital to visit us during weekdays. Our friends from Statesboro were amazing during this time, and worked out among themselves a schedule so that every weekend we had exactly one family set to visit as well. One memory, so clear in my mind, was a Friday night. Joe and Kristen, along with another friend Jodi, had come up to spend the weekend. We were sitting in the kitchen eating lasagna that someone had made, and I was soaking up the friendship and love of being in my own house with my friends, when the phone rang.

It was David, over at the hospital with Brian. He said, "This has been happening for a little while, I thought you'd want to hear this." I listened, and in the phone, I heard Brian! He was making a strange-sounding moan, but it didn't sound like he was in pain or distress. I had not heard sounds coming from him in weeks except for a few brief moments. David got back on the phone and said Brian had been making these sounds all evening, and that he didn't seem unhappy, it was more like he finally remembered how to make a sound come out on command. Despite how strange it sounded, I was crying tears of joy from finally hearing Brian's voice! All of our friends were amazed and happy to have been there to hear it as well.

During each weekday, Brian's schedule usually started around nine a.m. and ended around three p.m. He had a resting hour in the middle of the day, and at that time, he was still receiving his nutrition by g-tube, so he needed to be back in his bed for the hour it took for the formula to be pumped into his stomach. I went with him to every therapy, and learned techniques and options we could do back in the room to continue the rehab once we finished the formal schedule each day. One therapy that no one required, but that we took advantage of nearly daily, was the garden.

Even though it was the dead of winter, we were in Atlanta, so most days of January were still warm enough to spend time outside. I would bundle Brian up with a stocking hat, a couple of blankets, and down the elevator we could go, then out to the therapy garden provided by CHOA. Even in the winter, many vegetables and plants were growing, and I would try to help Brian smell the rosemary or the mint. There was a courtyard with a fountain, and we would sit and just watch the water and listen to the sounds. If planes went overhead, I pointed them out and talked to him about them. If we heard an ambulance, I would ask if he heard the siren. Every day I wheeled his chair up to some oversized animal sculptures, and say, "Do you see the turtle? What do turtles have on their backs? Shells!" and on and on. I was just trying to help him remember all the small little things that he had not been exposed to for all those weeks while he was in the coma. And honestly, I felt rejuvenated myself when I could get out of the four walls of his hospital room.

Brian's stay lasted one full month, and toward the end of that time, we began to make preparations for bringing him home. On a sunny day in late January, his physical and occupational therapists scheduled a time for them to conduct a site visit of our house, in order to make recommendations on what things we needed to be able to accommodate Brian. We were surprised to find out, Brian was going to go too!

First, a special child-seating expert brought us a modified car seat to go in the car to hold Brian. Since he was still unable to hold his head up at that time, it was designed much like an infant car seat, except many times bigger. They even made a small foam neck brace to place around his throat in order to help keep his neck from flopping forward. I can still remember the anxiety of us picking him out of his wheelchair and placing him in that seat. Yet as we drove the fifteen minutes back to our house, he seemed to enjoy the ride. He was calm, and seemed to be interested in the sights around him.

We pulled into the driveway. Earlier that morning, David had put up a poster that said "WELCOME HOME." This poster had been waiting for Ben earlier that month on his first day back to our house, now it welcomed Brian. The therapists were almost emotional when they saw this, and we reminded them, the last time Brian left this house was nearly two months prior. We made an awkward entry into the garage level of our split-level house. As the therapists checked out each room, and our completely un-wheelchair friendly floor plan, I expected they would have negative things to say.

Instead, they said we had some workable options, especially if we could get a ramp installed to our front porch so that the main living room and kitchen level of the house would be accessible. All the bedrooms and full bathrooms were on the top floor however, so they began to tell us they would recommend we place a hospital bed in the living room for Brian, and only carry him to the bathroom upstairs when two adults could be there. This was a rental property, and we imagined that we would definitely need to move when our lease was up, especially if Brian's recovery still meant he was wheelchair bound. But for the time being, we could adapt where we were.

Before leaving the house, I wheeled Brian into as many rooms as we could, and the final stop was the dining room. That happened to be where a huge toy cauldron from Halloween was sitting, which had been filled to the brim with candy the boys had collected just one month before the accident. Brian's eyes fixated on the candy bowl, and I can remember saying to him, "See, I didn't let Ben eat all your candy, Brian," and his response was totally apparent, even without words, he was a little boy excited to see his candy! Oh, these short little moments of something close to normalcy, we cherished them so much. We drove back to the hospital, and from then on, a spark came back into Brian's eyes, and it has never extinguished since. A few days later, we returned home for good.

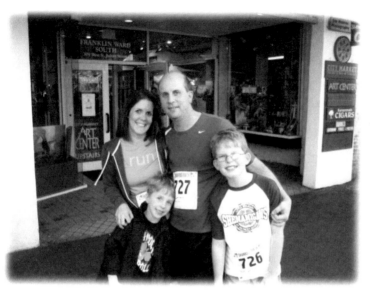

Our family running a 5K race six months before the accident.

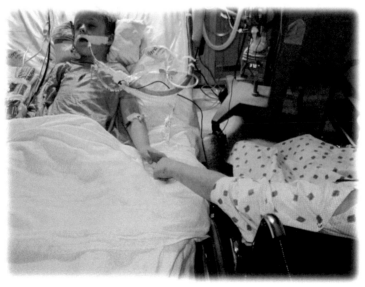

Before being transferred from the PICU, Ben says good-bye to Brian.

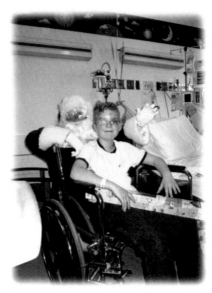

A surprise visit from "Santa" puts a little smile on Ben's face during his stay in the children's hospital.

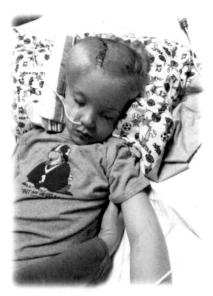

Brian with the ventilator removed two weeks after the accident. We expected this would be one of the last pictures we would have of him.

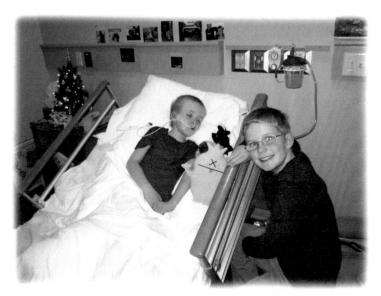

After praying for a miracle, Ben delivered a Christmas present to
Brian on Christmas Eve at the hospice. The swelling of Brian's
head had virtually disappeared overnight.

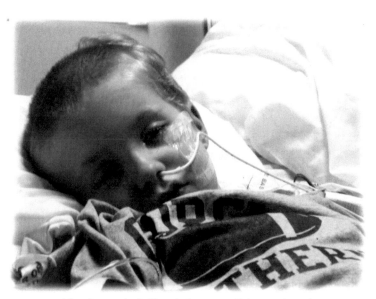

After three and a half weeks in a coma, Brian consistently
opened his eyes again as he began to recover.

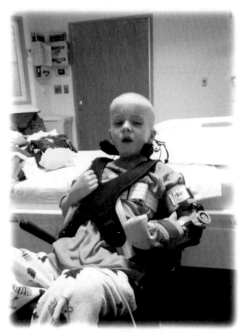

Beginning rehabilitation in Atlanta, first step was getting a wheelchair.

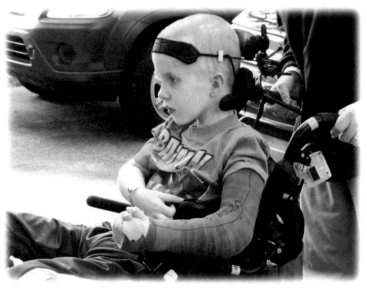

Brian's first visit home after nearly two months in the hospital.

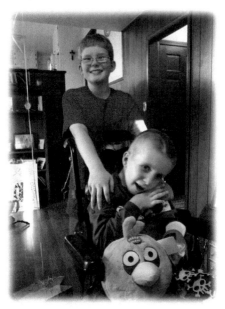

Both boys are all smiles as Brian returns home permanently.

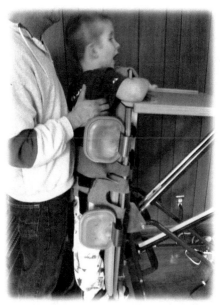

Home-based therapy was key; here David assists Brian in using the stander.

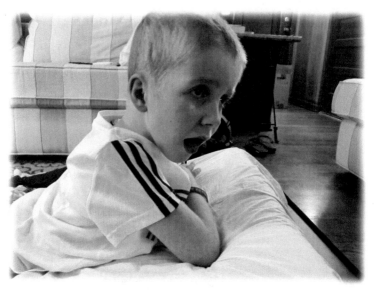

In late February, Brian had regained control of his head and neck, but still had little control of his body otherwise.

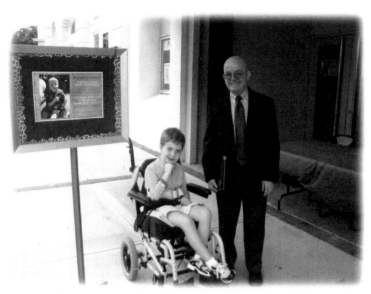

Brian with Dr. Michael Braz at one of the two benefit concerts held in April.

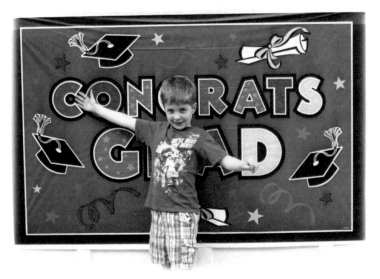

Brian graduates from the Day Rehabilitation program, June.

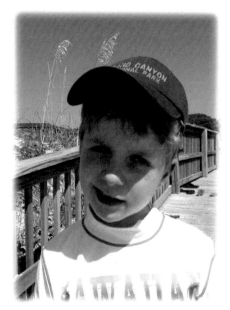

Enjoying a family vacation at the beach and feeling
grateful we could still have trips as a family.

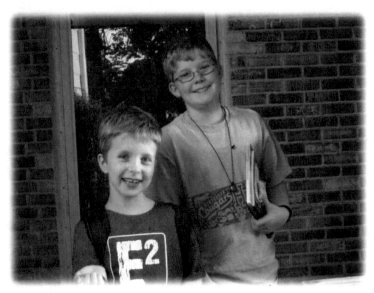

First day of school, 2012; Brian returns after a nine-month absence.

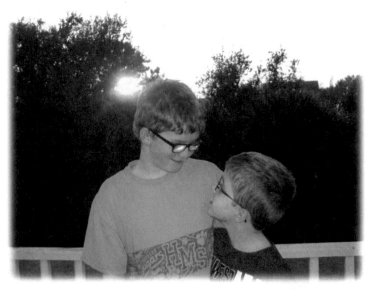

Brothers who love each other, one year after the accident.

Part Two:

Rehabilitation and Return to Real Life

I present these following chapters to you not in chronological order, but rather by themes. I couldn't begin to write (nor do I think it would be as interesting to read) a daily or weekly version of events, like I was able to do for our first two months following the accident. Instead, I have collected memories of several components of Brian's recovery, beginning with more details of his time at CHOA, then continuing with his outpatient therapies, his stay at the Day Rehabilitation program, and further. I have tried to share what the realities of this time were like in relation to each theme. Each chapter is told in chronological order, however, you will find each covers the months that followed in slightly different levels of detail, and each ends at slightly different points in time. This timeline shows the significant points of progress during these months.

2011

December 2	Accident occurs
December 3–19	Brian hospitalized in PICU, Savannah
December 19–27	Brian at Ogeechee Area Hospice, Statesboro
December 27–31	Brian re-admitted to PICU, Savannah

2012

January 1–6	Brian remains at PICU, Savannah
January 2	Cranioplasty (skull piece replaced)
January 4	G-tube surgery
January 6–February 7	Brian hospitalized at CHOA, Scottish Rite
Mid-February	Brian begins outpatient therapy
Late February	Brian begins to speak
Mid-March	Second Swallow Study conducted
March 23	Brian begins Day Rehab program
April 14	Benefit Concert in Statesboro; Brian's first overnight trip
May 9	Feeding tube removed
May 15	Brian walks independently for first time
June 20	Brian graduates Day Rehab
July 30	Third swallow study conducted
August 13	Brian returns to elementary school
October 14	Brian's eighth birthday

2013

January 10	Brian passes fourth and final swallow study
May 4	Brian completes 1K race at Evansdale Elementary
May 22	Brian receives awards at Honors Day, completes second grade

13

Walking

During Brian's stay at the CIRU, walking independently seemed like an impossible goal. We saw other kids there who were walking with help from the therapists. They all wore this industrial-looking, wide, white belt (a gait belt) so the therapist could have a hold on them for balance. We couldn't help but wonder if Brian would ever get to that point. He was eventually positioned in what is called an Eva walker. It was basically a walker with wheels (like you would see an elderly person use) except it had horizontal arm rests. In Brian's case, his arms couldn't really go on the arm rests properly because his biceps were still keeping his arms curled into a fetal type position. Nevertheless, when his physical therapist decided to pull him upright to standing and strap him into this thing, we finally got to see our boy "walking" again after six weeks.

It was tiring for him, and he was not verbal yet so he couldn't really communicate with us how it felt, but I could see in his eyes that it was extremely tough. One therapist would stand behind him while another scooted along backwards on a rolling short stool, helping to lift and position his legs and move them forward. It was a two-person job. *How in the world would we ever be able to do this once we left the hospital?* I thought to myself.

Once he started this element of therapy, he did begin to show some improvements. At that time, his right leg was extremely tight and rigid, but his left leg could bend and he soon was picking that leg up and taking a step (still with a lot of help from the therapists or me). The right leg we had to manually lift every time. Imagine if you were flexing your thigh muscle and straightening your leg out as far as you can. This is how Brian's right leg stayed during much of his time inpatient. It was another side effect of the injury in the brain, and so odd for us to get our heads around the fact that the actual muscles and bones of his legs and arms weren't injured in the crash, yet he had such limited use of them.

When he did "walk" we cheered and gave him encouragement for going a little bit farther than the time before. I kept telling the therapists about how competitive Brian is and how athletic. We would use visual cues like the tile of the floor changing color to motivate him and give him a "finish line." How much that helped him we will never know, since he could not tell us how he was feeling. But it gave me a semblance of normalcy to think my little boy was still in there being motivated by something like finishing a race.

As the hospital came close to discharging Brian, we were given confusing and somewhat frustrating information about how to get a similar piece of equipment for our house. Even though the rental property we lived in had a split-level design and, therefore, wasn't going to be easy to navigate entirely, we did have a pretty large level with kitchen, dining room, and living room that we thought we could use to help Brian continue walking. I still to this day cannot completely understand the process that occurred (or more accurately, didn't occur) to try to get our health insurance to purchase a walker for Brian.

By late February, we were advised by Brian's physical therapist that the best equipment to help him gain strength in his legs and move toward walking again someday would be a stander. This is a huge machine with a level board that can be raised or lowered to hold patients upright. Brian used one in CIRU and it was helping him bear weight on his feet and gain strength in his legs. It requires two people to get the patient onto it most of the time. Not only is it expensive (several thousand dollars typically), apparently it is rare that insurance will agree to pay for it. Yet again, our journey was guided by divine intervention ... Though it should no longer be a surprise that God was working through human beings here on earth to achieve the miracle of Brian's recovery, it still was shocking to us by how blatant his control was over situations that were helping us on the path to recovery.

The physical therapist had one last suggestion before we made the purchase of the expensive equipment. She directed us to an organization that provides used medical equipment to families in need. We called, but were told the equipment we sought wouldn't be available for weeks. Eager to help Brian get closer to walking, we decided to go ahead and just make the purchase and figured it was a good use of some very generous donations people had made to an account set up to help Brian. It is hard to accurately convey how urgently we felt about helping our child make progress.

The frustrating and slow system of insurance and medical equipment ordering is not the point of this story, but it is accurate to say we felt we *had* to act, for Brian's sake; he couldn't put off this part of his recovery for months. In retrospect, it was clear that most medical professionals had a pretty pessimistic view of his chance of a speedy recovery, and therefore were not necessarily overly concerned with timeframes like two to three months to get equipment. I mean, if the kid was unlikely to ever get out of the wheelchair anyway, what was another couple of months? That was *never* our view, we had a picture in our head of him walking, running, being independent again. We made the order for the equipment one day around three p.m.

At five thirty p.m. the phone rang, David answered, and it was a local minister who told us that his church had been praying for us for two months. Out of the blue that day, he felt he needed to give us a call to let us know his church would like to do anything they could to help us, financially or otherwise. David said, "Actually, the one thing Brian needs right now is a stander." The pastor offered to purchase it for us, but also asked if we'd contacted the organization I mentioned above. David explained how far we were on the wait list, and that it seemed unlikely. The minister said he knew the director of that organization and would give them a call to check. If not, they would buy us the stander!

When David came up to tell me, "Guess what? We don't have to worry about buying the stander," and explained what had happened, I just started crying. God kept stepping in just at the right time and providing. I mean, literally on the same day. Just like the day back in late January that the therapists told us we needed a hospital bed for Brian once he came home from the hospital (rather than just moving his regular bed to the living room to make it more accessible as we had planned). *That same day*, we got an e-mail from some neighbors (whom we'd never met). The wife said her mother had recently passed, and she and her dad wondered if we could possibly use a hospital bed and some other medical equipment they were about to donate. It's difficult to believe these "coincidences" and yet, they really happened. That night we looked at each other and said, "Guess God really wants Brian to have a stander!"

The next day we actually received a call from the organization who said they *did* have a stander for us; we could pick it up that day. We arranged for my sister Bridget (who had selflessly come to help us out for nearly a month) to stay with the boys and we headed down to the warehouse (about thirty minutes away). En route the minister called, "Hey, I sure would love to see Brian, and by the way, I have a pickup and I could meet you down there and bring it back for you." So that is exactly what we did. His son was also a first grader at the boys' school Evansdale Elementary and, though not in Brian's class, knew Brian from the playground. They came over and got the stander set up, visited with Brian, prayed with us, and also offered to make him an honorary member of the first grade little league team at their church. We told the minister, "Thank you so much for 'deciding' to call us that day . . . although we think someone else helped you make that decision!" We got Brian in the stander the next day, and prayed eventually those legs would be ready to hold up his body all the time.

We had the equipment we thought would be the key, and we began to try to use it. Unfortunately, we did not expect Brian to have such a negative reaction when using the stander. He would cry and scream, despite trying to distract him with videos, books, games, or anything we could, he rarely made it more than twenty minutes in the thing. One friend who came by and saw it in our den said, "It looks like a torture device!" (not in front of Brian thankfully) and he wasn't wrong. Patients stand by having their arms and legs secured with big Velcro straps, and then other straps wrap around the torso to hold that upright as well. Yet, we were determined to try to get him in the stander daily, and did the best we could. Meanwhile, as he was gaining some strength in his abdomen and core, we were able to start a much more enjoyable option—holding him upright under his arms and "walking" him around the house. At first, he had his feet on top of our feet, like you would do with a toddler just learning to walk. Eventually he was able to begin to move his own legs in order to take some steps.

From the time he was hospitalized to the subsequent months, a change had occurred in the function of Brian's legs. Initially his right leg was stiff and inflexible while his left leg could bend and he could show some control of movement. Eventually his left hamstring began to tighten and his ankles bend. While he gained strength and flexibility on the right, the left side was weaker and he had much less ability to use it (even in the stander, his left foot wouldn't go flat due to the stretch required in the hamstring and ankle to do that). It is something I wish we could have addressed earlier; however, the sheer quantity of things we were trying to "fix" meant that we just had to prioritize and do the best we could.

In mid-March we had an appointment scheduled with a special office of CHOA to determine what size wheelchair should be ordered for Brian to have as his permanent chair. As a patient at CHOA, he was given a loaner chair that was sent home with him at discharge; however it was not meant for him to keep, partially because while they were refurbished, these chairs were not new, and also because it would be better to have a chair built that would fit his exact physical specifications more closely. When this appointment was scheduled for Brian in late January, they said it would be best to wait until March, by then we'd know more of his long-term prognosis.

Around the time this appointment was scheduled, Brian's physical therapist suggested we ask the specialists at the wheelchair fitting office to also provide measurements for what size of gait trainer would be the best for him. A gait trainer is a walker that incorporates a sling type seat to help support the patient initially, and then can be removed later as a person is able to hold his or her own body weight. It was proposed this would really be the best option for Brian, and could replace the stander as a mechanism to hold him upright (this sounded great to us, given his reaction to the stander).

We wheeled Brian into a room filled to the brim with child-sized medical equipment (if you wanted to ever see a sad sight, imagining that many children needing walkers, standers, wheelchairs, etc., will do it). The therapists measured him, brought out a sample gait trainer, strapped him in, and I watched as my child, with their help, used it to *walk out of the room!* Brian's determination and strength were on full display, and while it wasn't an easy process by any means, he made it work. As he and the therapist came back in the room, I heard some of the best news I could imagine. They said based on the amazing recovery he was making, they would *not* be ordering him a permanent wheelchair at this time, and told me to keep the one he had.

No one would make real predictions about his chances of regaining function again, but I could tell by their reaction and their insistence that he was not a candidate for a permanent wheelchair fitting; they thought he had a chance. We did agree to put the request through to our insurance to purchase this gait trainer for him, though I was warned the process is often bogged down and it would be a long wait. It was no matter; the best news was the wheelchair might not be forever. Deep in my heart, I had believed this all along, and it had spurred us to take the actions we did. Finally, we'd been affirmed in thinking this was really possible!

Brian began his day rehabilitation program at the end of March, and he was able to use a gait trainer and other equipment daily while there. We saw progress every week, not only in his legs, but also in his overall strength and stamina. We continued to "walk" him around the house by holding him under his arms, and it was gratifying to see how more and more of his own control was coming back, especially in moving his legs. A huge benefit to his ability to "walk" with our help was getting him up and down the stairs in our home. As mentioned, we were renting a split-level home, and while we were able to set up a hospital bed for Brian in our living room that was accessible from the outside by a ramp built for us by friends, there was no bathroom on that level. It required David carrying Brian and me following behind to spot them to get him up the stairs for baths. This was "do-able," although hard on our backs as Brian has always been a big and tall boy for his age—at this point, he was well over sixty pounds. By him being able to stay upright while we helped him walk up or down the stairs, we could finally stop carrying him every time he needed a bath.

Around this same time, we were finally able to allow him to stay in his bedroom. The hospital bed sat in the living room for a couple more months, until we finally returned it to the generous family who'd given it to us in the first place. I sometimes still envision that bed up in the corner of the living room and remember the many nights I slept across the room from Brian on the sofa, waking to help him in the night, and living a surreal life of hospital equipment filling our home. The night we put Brian to bed in his own bedroom (with Spider-Man sheets and his books and toys surrounding him), I said a prayer thanking God for that tiny bit of normalcy we had regained. It was something any parent would take for granted, seeing their child asleep in his bed, yet we felt such joy in that simple sight. It had been more than three months since we'd seen it, and thinking about the nights we'd gone to sleep never knowing if we'd see it again, we were filled with gratitude.

Brian worked at his day rehabilitation on strengthening his core as well, and eventually could roll himself over and sit up on his own. Throughout April, we saw him make gains, and he could finally sit in a chair or on the couch (instead of his wheelchair) when inside the house. But the day in early May when he was finally able to stand up from sitting by himself still caught us a little bit by surprise. Luckily, we videotaped the moment, and it's still sweet to watch it. Brian used his right leg and foot to hold his weight and stood up. You can hear Ben in the background, as usual making Brian laugh. After I said, "He's standing up!" Ben yelled out "By himself!" in a funny voice. Brian loves to watch this video, I think to hear his brother, but I love seeing the joy and happiness on his face when he was able to do what had been so long impossible for him—standing on his own. His left leg was still weaker, the muscles tight, the hamstring drawing his leg up in a slight bend, but no matter. He was standing!

It was a rapid progression from that point to two weeks later when Brian made his first few steps across the den completely on his own. Again, thank goodness we had the camera close so we could document the exact moment, it is a victory that was five months in the making. Much like a toddler who cruises next to the couch, he started off right next to the sofa for some balance, but the next thing you know he was walking right across the room. Landing in the chair, he was smiling and responded to our excitement with a laugh. From that day forward, there hasn't been a day that Brian didn't walk again on his own two feet at least some, with his strength and balance improving dramatically.

I was able to talk with his physical therapist at his day rehab program around this same time, and tell her the news. Due to regulations and to prevent falls, while he was there he had to have his gait belt on, and have a therapist holding it, so he hadn't been able to freely walk without another person yet at rehab. Her advice to me though was this, "Cancel the order for that gait trainer; he's already past it!" Yes, the gait trainer we'd ordered back in late March was *still* not in by mid-May, and yet, through God's grace and Brian's work, he'd already surpassed the need for it. Thank goodness we were able to make that call, and the equipment never arrived. Even though insurance would have paid for it, we were still grateful to be able to cancel that order.

Brian continued to make progress throughout the summer, even as he transitioned from the day rehab program to returning to his physical therapy in an outpatient capacity. We spent as much time as we could with him in our neighborhood pool, where the water helped him with balance and he could stretch the muscles in his legs and begin to be steadier on his feet. As the summer came to a close and we prepared for his return to elementary school, we all agreed he had enough balance and control to attend school without the help of any walker or wheelchair.

One day, I packed the boys up in the van, hoisted that loaner wheelchair from the hospital up into the back as I'd done a couple hundred times before, and drove a few miles up the road to the medical equipment store. As I mentioned, this chair had been on loan, and had obviously belonged to a girl named Arteshia before it was lent out to Brian (based on the fact that her name was stenciled on the seat of the chair itself). As we drove, I worried that Brian would have a negative reaction to us returning the wheelchair; though he was able to walk on his own two feet by this point, his stamina was low and he sometimes asked us to let him have the chair when he just didn't have the energy to walk. Despite this, we felt it would do Brian good and ultimately motivate him by returning it. (Meanwhile, we did have a much less cumbersome transport wheelchair that we kept knowing there would still be instances where we may need to help him cover larger distances.)

Ben almost instinctively knew that Brian was showing signs of becoming upset by the loss of the wheelchair, and began a running joke similar to the now-overused jokes like "The eighties called, they want their hairstyle back." Ben said to Brian "Hey . . . guess what? Arteshia called . . . she wants her chair back!" It was enough to break the tension, and Brian laughed at his brother and promptly retold that same joke once we were inside the store to the lady helping us. She may not have gotten it, but for me, seeing Ben and Brian cutting jokes and laughing together while that chair was wheeled away was incredible.

The first day of school came. We had prepared Brian's teachers, paraprofessional, principal, and special education liaison that he would need to be accompanied at all times, and was still at risk for falls in his current state. Their readiness for him to return was heartwarming, and while our decision for him to go this way was riskier, in the end, he made a more normal transition back to the classroom, and eventually was really quite independent while at school. I couldn't help but reflect on how far he had come when that first day of school actually arrived.

 . . . [E]ven with the positive approach here in Atlanta, in rehabilitation circles language was always couched with "if" and "might" and "maybe someday." As in, "Maybe someday he would be able to return to a school setting for children with disabilities and in wheelchairs and/or other severe impairments." Impossible to think he might actually walk his own legs through the hallway to sit down at his regular old second grade desk, unpack his regular old second grade supplies, and get on with the rest of his life. Except that's exactly what Brian Murkison did today.

It would be wonderful to say that was the happy ending, and that he just easily regained his ability to walk perfectly after that point. But the path of rehabilitation from brain injury is not that smooth, and struggles still laid ahead for our boy.

About a month into the school year, a process of progressive casting began to stretch Brian's ankles into a more neutral position. Brain injury can cause certain muscles to receive constant signal to fire, while other muscles cannot receive a similar signal. In Brian's case, the hamstring, calf, and ankle, particularly on his left side, were tight and he could not fully extend his heel to the floor. When he walked, the ball of his left foot would touch down, but not the heel, giving him an unbalanced gait and noticeable limp. The casts went on to both feet and were to be changed out each week, stretching him each time to a more and more neutral positioning of the feet.

During this period, Brian participated in a walk-a-thon fundraiser for his school where the children walked the athletic field and were given prizes for the number of laps completed. Even with both feet in walking casts, he completed three laps that day. We felt such pride for him, and yet, our boy the year before would have *run*, not walked . . . would have finished ten laps, not three. In the constant roller coaster of emotions that go with a TBI recovery, moments were often bittersweet in this way.

As the casting process continued, however, we began to see Brian showing signs of severe emotional distress. Combined with the pressures of being back in a classroom for the first time in nine months, his behavior became erratic and sometimes aggressive. We had read about this in the TBI literature, but had really not seen Brian "acting out" in such a way until the casts went on. After a few weeks of this (and before the proposed end date of the process), we went to the doctors and said, "Something needs to change." The team agreed to discontinue the casting process at that point to help with his emotional challenges, but was happy to report the process *had* done some of what it was intended to do. Brian's ankle on his left side was now at a point that he had enough range for a permanent leg brace, which could be worn inside his shoe and would be less invasive and irritating for him.

We soon found ourselves watching as Brian began to progress in walking up and down stairs by himself, being able and willing to walk the one third of a mile to school some mornings, and ultimately, by the end of the school year, we had yet another emotional and rewarding milestone. Each spring our elementary school hosted a 1K and 5K walk/run as a fundraiser. Brian and David trained for several weeks, walking the course of the 1K route, preparing for Brian's participation in his first race since the accident. The morning came for the race, and instead of a typical Georgia May morning of warm sun and blue skies, it was a chilly, cold, and rainy morning. Never mind that. Brian was determined, and his determination inspired us all. With his grandparents and me by his side (and his dad staying back to video and photograph the whole thing), Brian completed the 1K route in around nineteen minutes. Those who knew him were cheering loudly as he finished, and the little competitor in him was back. A long way from his "races" in the hospital while three adults held him and "walked" him. A miraculously long way . . .

14

Eating

When Brian was a little boy, we were always amazed at the variety and amount of food he would eat. As a toddler, he would happily eat pork roast, vegetables, or casserole. He learned how to use the sign language symbol for "more" before he began to talk, and would almost always give us the little "pat-pat" hand gesture of his fingers coming together to tell us he wanted more to eat. We even made up a family tradition of singing a song to him to the tune of the theme song of Winnie the Pooh.

 Bottomless Pit . . . Bottomless Pit. He eats and eats and eats and eats and eats and eats and eats and eats. Bottomless Pit . . . Bottomless Pit. Brian could eat all day (or all night . . . or all weekend).

It was just a fun, silly tradition in our family. As he grew, Brian continued to have a diverse palate. Often he used it very much to his advantage. Ben has always been a fairly picky eater, and we would struggle to get him to even try new things. I can remember one night in particular when Brian was only maybe three or four. The vegetable of the night was broccoli. Brian put his broccoli on his fork, shoved it in his mouth, looked right at Ben and said, "Mom, your broccoli is delicious!" (Take that, big brother . . .) As he got a little older, he would even want to try ethnic cuisine like Thai noodles, even asking to go to the local Thai restaurant for his birthday, pretty unusual for a five-year-old.

That's why it was so heartrending to see him unable to eat at all for so many weeks following the accident. Initially, patients in the hospital have a tube placed into their stomach through their nose. For the first three weeks after the accident, he received a formula through his tube, fed drip by drip from a pump alongside his bed. Although some medical staff encouraged us to remove this during the period in which everyone thought Brian was too far gone to recover, we refused. To this day, I am so grateful we didn't listen to anyone asking us to consider that option. Even as we moved him to a hospice, where in essence we expected he would pass at any time, he still received nutrition and water via this method.

It was only after returning to Memorial when the miracle began to play out that the doctors and we made the choice to move forward with a laparoscopic procedure to place a g-tube port into Brian's stomach. The surgery was very low risk, and it allowed him to receive the same nutrient filled formula directly into his stomach, removing the intrusive tube from his nose.

At the point this surgery occurred, we were still shell-shocked. We knew this step was a recommendation usually only made for patients who were expected to survive, and for that, we were so thankful. However, the pessimism by the medical team of Brian's ultimate ability to recover fully was still strong. It was evidenced so clearly on the day of the surgery. The gastroenterologist who was going to do the procedure came and asked David if we had any questions. "Yes, how difficult will it be to remove this port at the point Brian can eat again on his own?" The doctor looked at David and said, "If by some miracle he is ever able to get rid of this, it's not hard to remove." If by some miracle . . . after all we'd been through by that point, hearing something like that was hard to take.

We were forced to imagine the prediction of Brian never having the physical capacity to eat again as a real possibility. During the initial dire predictions given to us, a concern that he had lost his ability to swallow or have a gag reflex was very real. The brainstem handles these critical functions, and this was where doctors thought too much damage had already occurred to ever heal. You don't consciously tell yourself to swallow hundreds of times throughout the day; your brain just tells the throat and mouth to do their thing. If you get something in your windpipe by drinking it too fast, you don't consciously decide to cough, it just happens. These critical functions were expected to be lost forever. As difficult as that was to hear, we looked at the g-tube surgery as a step in the road, and tried not to think the worst.

Luckily, we met with much more optimism and a plan of recovery once we arrived at CHOA. Within the first week, speech therapists began to work with Brian to engage him in stimulating the muscles in his mouth. Brain injury is often coupled with the actual occurrence of, or at least the symptoms of, a stroke. In fact, the left side of Brian's face was droopy, he did not have the ability to keep his mouth closed, and it hung open often in an expression that is best described as slack-jawed. How would we move from this to a kid who is eating hot dogs and popcorn and apples and Thai food?

The speech therapists began to introduce ice chips for Brian to try to swallow. That seemed to be moderately successful, so they moved on to a small bit of yogurt, then applesauce, or shavings off a popsicle. As a positive incentive, he was offered a lick of a lollipop. It's so sad to remember in those days before he could communicate, we had to just speak to him and hope he understood us. Seeing him getting a taste of the sugary sucker was both profound and heartbreaking. Because a seven-year-old boy having a piece of candy is about as natural a sight as you can get, and here he was, only being able to have it placed in his mouth by someone else.

Nevertheless, he did begin to make progress in swallowing. It was explained to us that they always begin with thick substances like pudding, because it is easiest to stay all together as it passes the windpipe. Water or liquids, however, are the hardest. Water's molecules don't bind closely together like a pudding, so as a patient attempts to swallow, it's much harder to control where all the parts of the water are going. A special product called a thickener was used to turn liquids into more of a syrup consistency. He began practicing with thickened apple juice and chocolate milk, using a straw to suck. It was actually amazing what he was able to accomplish during those first four weeks at the rehab unit, considering where he started.

Near the end of our time in the hospital, the speech therapist explained to me that they needed to do something called a swallow study on Brian. They could see that he was getting these small bits of food down, but they couldn't be sure if it was going into his stomach or (dangerously) into his wind pipe and down into his lungs. Because no one knew for certain if he had the ability to respond physically when something went down the wrong way, it was a real concern. Food getting into his lungs would likely cause him to develop pneumonia or other lung issues.

The speech therapist and I wheeled Brian to the Radiology department. A special booster seat was set up to prop him in, as he could still not sit on his own. As the speech therapist gave Brian sips of juice, then thickened juice, then bites of the pudding and yogurt laced with barium, a radiologist watched in real-time to see where exactly the food was going. The test is done in a way that once any sign of food going down the wrong way is detected, they stop that type in order to not cause harm to the patient just for the sake of the test. Results showed he was able to swallow the soft food and the thickened liquid, but the regular liquid was still a problem. The thought of our little boy having to go through life always carrying a packet of thickening agent with him in order to drink something was so sad. I bring up these fears as a way to show that while we still believed in him, and had faith in what God could accomplish, it was a battle every day to not let fears and worries like that take over.

As we were sent home from the hospital, and began outpatient speech therapy, we helped Brian practice eating every day. The amounts were so small; but his nutrition still came from the six boxes of formula that we sent through his feeding tube every day. Part of our training before coming home with him involved learning how to operate and troubleshoot the pump that pushed the formula through his tube. It was delivered originally over the course of an hour, and then a slower drip over the course of several hours at night. This time period became really challenging as we started his outpatient therapies however. He was supposed to get an hour of feeding drip at eight a.m., twelve p.m., and four p.m. You can't be driving or in transit during any of those times. Meanwhile, he was supposed to be in therapies sometimes two hours at a time, five days a week. Managing the timing of the feeding pump was no small issue. As he could not swallow well, all of his many medications were also delivered via the tube. This meant we had to crush (and mix with water) several medications a day, and then insert them using a syringe into the tube. For weeks we crushed pills, mixed them in tiny cups, then washed and dried cups and syringes over and over. It may seem small, but somehow the tedium of all those little steps was really heartbreaking sometimes.

As the weeks went by, he began to show real progress. At therapy, he was given a small bit of graham cracker. This was considered safe for him because it would soften into a consistency like pudding as it sat in his mouth. He struggled to have enough muscle strength in his mouth to clear all the food out however. Eventually his therapist even made him a special placemat that showed a little boy eating, then sticking his tongue out covered in food, then swallowing to remind Brian to always clear his mouth.

By late March, all the therapists and doctors decided it was time for Brian to begin the Day Rehab program operated through CHOA. He would be gone from nine to three daily, and would receive all of the therapies he'd been doing as outpatient during his time there each day. In preparation for him beginning the program, another swallow study was scheduled. We had seen him progress so much by that time, and were so ready to hear that he had passed the test and could move back into eating and drinking regular food.

It was a huge disappointment when he did not pass. Our expectations were crushed, and at the time, it was easy to fall into a huge pit of self-pity and despair. Voices in my head said, "See, he isn't going to get any better." For about two days, I believed it. I was sullen and somewhat frustrated on Brian's first speech therapy visit following the results. But to my surprise, his therapist was happy. She told me that his responses were better than had been seen originally, that he *was* making progress, and that even though the "thin" or regular liquids were still out of reach, he could begin to add more normal food to his diet. It was a huge lesson in not letting fear and despair drag me down. I took her enthusiasm, and ran with it. We began to re-introduce all kinds of foods to Brian from a list provided by the doctors. Very quickly after he started at Day Rehab, the doctors agreed the amount of nutrition he could (and did) eat on his own could replace the need for him to have those hour-long feedings three times a day. Taking away the imposition of three hours of his day and getting his feedings while he slept made a huge difference in his ability to recover in so many other ways! It was a beautiful turning point in his recovery.

While at Day Rehab, a new set of speech therapists began to work with Brian. They began to practice giving him distilled, purified water to practice swallowing non-thickened liquids. The amounts were small, and everyone had to be very careful to have cleaned his mouth out first so that the risk of anything getting into his lungs was minimized. We were given permission to do this at home as well, and so began David and Brian's morning tradition of trying to take sips of water from his Spider-Man cup. The cup had a lid with a straw built in, if it tipped over not much spilled. And Brian responded pretty well to being able to get this level of swallowing figured out.

About halfway through his time at Day Rehab, Brian began to ask his nurse why he had to have his medicine put into his tube. She asked him "Do you think you can swallow a pill?" and Brian said he wanted to try. Sure enough, he easily made the transition, and the medical professionals gave us the approval to stop using his g-tube for his medication, and to allow him to take it by mouth. Luckily, the number of medications he was taking by this point had begun to drop, and it was really not as cumbersome (or frequent) as it had been.

We also kept logs of the amounts and types of food Brian was eating daily. The medical staff thought he was getting sufficient calories based on our list, but they submitted this log to a nutritionist to be sure. When the report came back that he was consuming enough calories with the food he was eating, the amazing milestone that the gastroenterologist back in Savannah said would probably never come, actually happened. On a Tuesday in early May, the nurse called and told me, "We took Brian's g-tube port out today. He may be a little sore, but it will close up in a couple of days, and he did great." Sure enough, when Brian came home on the bus from Day Rehab that day the very first thing he did was show off his "second belly button," where the port had come out of his stomach. I asked him what it was like when the doctor had taken it out and he said, "I thought it would hurt, but she took it out and then I said, 'Was that all?' because it didn't hurt at all." We just couldn't wait to share this great news with our friends and family, and we all celebrated together in amazement at what a few months of recovery had brought.

As the three months of Day Rehab came to a close, again, the therapists thought he had likely conquered this swallowing of regular water difficulty, and a third swallow study was scheduled. By now, we *really* felt like he would pass. We'd seen him gain such ease with the thickened liquids, he had never developed any lung issue that would indicate some of these things were going down the wrong way, and his general health and strength of his muscles was so much stronger. On top of all of this, he was about to go back to school, and be in a setting where having to drink a special drink was going to be much more difficult. We were so prayerful and hopeful the day of the test. However, one drink in, and he failed it. I cannot tell you how sickening the feeling was to see that image on the screen of his water going down slightly into his windpipe. Worse, during this and all of the other exams, when that occurred, he never coughed, never showed he had the reflex to protect himself. I cannot say during the time since we began his rehabilitation there were many days worse than these two swallow study days.

During these times of disappointment, you want to scream, cry, and make someone tell you *why is this happening!* But what you really do is keep it together somehow, thank the speech therapist for her time, smile at Brian, and say, "You did a great job, honey! We're just going to keep working on this a little longer," and you move on. After this third test, David and I really did begin to believe that it was possible that he would always have to adapt his lifestyle to thicken any beverage he wanted to drink. It was about six months into the process by this point, and honestly, it had become very much second nature. So in the car there were always five or six packets of thickener, just in case we needed them. When we went out to eat, the last question we always asked ourselves was, "Do we have thickener and a cup for Brian?" and we just went from there. At school each day, I sent Brian's lunch with a container of thickened apple juice, and his teacher knew to let me know if the class had a party or was going to be drinking something outside of lunch so I could get his fixed up. It really did become routine, and the fall progressed.

We had a doctor's visit in mid-December to assess where he was in recovery, adjust medications, and schedule further treatments. One thing the doctor said was that he wanted Brian to do another swallow study. About five months had passed by this point, and the doctor was optimistic based on Brian's continued improved health and strength that he would have gained the muscle coordination in his mouth and throat muscles needed to pass it. So one morning in January, we arrived at the hospital.

Unlike the other times, I actually felt myself believing it probably wasn't going to be a passing test. I guess I just tried to block my fears by being pessimistic in the first place. As we sat in the waiting room, I simply prayed a silent prayer that God would help me deal with the results. A therapist Brian had known from his Day Rehab time was on duty that morning, and came out with a huge smile and a hug for Brian. "Come on, Brian, let's go see if you pass this test!" she said. Off we went, me trailing behind pessimistically like a dark storm cloud, the two of them happily chattering and catching up. Since he was already cleared for food and thickened liquids, they really only planned to try the thin liquids to minimize his radiation exposure.

Drink one, I really could almost not look (in fact, I don't actually remember if I did). But I heard the therapist say, "Good job, Brian, let's try one more." I knew from the previous tests, if they see evidence it's not going down right, they stop. Now, I was watching closely, and as the water went in his mouth, his throat muscles moved, and down it all went, right where it was supposed to go! The therapist said, "Okay, thanks!" and I was literally lost for a minute. What did she mean? She must have realized by my confused face and said, "He passed! I'll get the report written up for the doctors, but he's cleared for any food of drink." We have had many proud moments during Brian's recovery, but this one was as poignant as any other.

I couldn't wait to let David know, and Brian was so proud of the news! One thing that he was really excited about was finally getting to switch to the hot meals at school and to be able to stop bringing his lunch every day. We stopped at a store on the way home so he could pick out a prize, and he wanted a smiley face balloon as well (which of course I bought for him). That night when we got home, I threw the container of powdered thickener in the trashcan and posted a picture of it. The memory of that smiley face balloon, and the sight of the then unnecessary thickening powder still brings a smile to my face. To celebrate, that night we let Brian pick the restaurant and we went out to eat (pizza, no surprise), and for the first time in over a year, our kid was finally able to order a root beer in a cup and drink it, without any modifications. As a parent, you cannot begin to know the relief and happiness this simple action caused. The big smile on his face said it all, and it was beautiful.

15

The Role of Music

Brian sat in his wheelchair. His arms were caged in metallic braces designed to help keep his arms from curling inward to the fetal position (a side effect of the brain injury called posturing). His head was strapped to a headrest with a band of black cloth, preventing him from bobbing his head forward like a newborn baby. The music therapist positioned herself directly in Brian's eyesight and began to play her guitar and sing. She would sing a few bars of popular songs that Brian knew and then stop, in essence, giving him a chance to keep going with the song. Except he couldn't. He couldn't even make a sound, much less sing along with her. As sad of a scene as this was, we were grateful that the hospital provided music therapy to Brian, because we knew how important music had always been to him, and hoped maybe, just maybe, it would help him break through.

Every couple of days we would get music therapy added to his schedule. And slowly over time, he began to show signs he was aware. A small move of his arm or leg, a glance when the therapist asked him questions. I did my best to remember songs that Brian had liked before the accident. It hit me one day that he liked a song called "Tonight, Tonight." I could remember him upstairs in his bedroom singing it at the top of his lungs one day before the accident, and it made me laugh by how enthusiastic he was. I had to Google it to figure out what song it was, but once I did, I told the therapist and she said she'd add it in. A part of the chorus to the song goes "La, la, la . . . whatever. La, la, la . . . it doesn't matter."

I will never forget the day that Brian was listening to his therapist play that song for him, and all of a sudden, I saw his tongue start to move to the top of his mouth when she sang "La, la, la." He was attempting to make an "L"! We both saw him do it, and she stopped and cheered for him to do it again. It is really hard to capture the significance of this moment. It had been weeks since we had seen anything like a purposeful verbal response from Brian, weeks since we'd heard his voice. And even though he couldn't make sounds yet, seeing that tongue trying to work so he could sing along to a song he loved gave so much hope. We could see the glimmers of him coming back to us because of a catchy pop song.

A friend and colleague read about this on our blog and was compelled to try to share this story with the band itself, a group from Nashville called Hot Chelle Rae. She searched the Internet for their contact information and wrote their manager, retelling the story and asking if the band could send Brian a get-well card. Much to our surprise a few days later, my friend forwarded a video message that had been filmed of the band members talking to Brian, encouraging him to get better and thanking him for liking their song so much. They even invited him to come to a concert the next time they were in Atlanta. I admit it was a feel-good moment, and a bit of a rush to get this type of attention for Brian. But at the time, it was a ridiculous notion to think he could go to a concert, just another reminder that our life was just so entirely different than it used to be. When a short three months later the band did actually come to Atlanta, they were true to their word, and provided us a chance to come and meet the band and attend the concert. It was surprising how long Brian lasted, given at that time he was usually in bed by seven-thirty or eight p.m. not to mention the volume a concert like this produces. I brought a whole case of earplugs (which he kept taking out) to try to keep the stimulation from being too much. Brian made it long enough during the headliner's show to hear his favorite song before we had to make our exit. Still, if you had told me back at the hospital we'd have been able to do any part of that night, I would have had a hard time believing it.

Music continued to play a part in Brian's recovery through the actions of several friends from our former hometown of Statesboro. A retired music professor, Dr. Michael Braz, had been a follower of our blog and our Facebook page. He had known David back in his high school days, and had worked with Ben during a summer theater camp a couple of years before. One day, out of the blue, Dr. Braz e-mailed us with an idea. He wanted to have a concert and help our family by raising money for our medical costs and expenses. At first we were unsure, and didn't feel we should ask others for this type of support. It was difficult finding yourself in the role of the "needy" after so many years of trying to find ways to help those in need. Finally, after praying about it, we agreed to have the concert as a celebration of the miracle that God had given us in healing Brian. We determined we would take a portion of the proceeds and make contributions to the Ogeechee Area Hospice and the Ronald McDonald house, the two non-profits that had made such an impact in keeping our family comfortable during the worst times.

The date was set and another family friend, Lori Grice, a well-known photographer with strong connections in the Statesboro business community, began to provide the marketing, planning, and organizing of volunteers it took to make the event so special. She and her husband, DeWayne, collected items for a silent auction, arranged for the theater to host the event, and handled everything down to printing posters and flyers to advertise. Friends and family in Statesboro sold advance tickets, and the excitement grew. It was our plan to bring Brian and Ben to the concert in Statesboro, but it was a nerve-wracking idea because it would be the first time we had left home overnight with Brian since the accident.

The day of the concert came, and Brian was excited. The concert itself was so inspirational, with Dr. Braz playing requests along with many popular tunes on the piano. We sat in the front row, and had our closest friends right behind us. As I turned around to see nearly the entire theater full of people, my heart was just full of gratitude. I just felt an overwhelming sense that we had chosen to do the right thing by coming, because these were the people who had prayed with us, grieved with us, and then began to have hope with us. They were part of this miracle too, and by bringing the boys to a celebration filled with music, we were allowing them to share in our joy. Some of the most special people in the audience were the Air Evac crew that had transported Brian by helicopter that first night, as well as Tyler Thompson, who had called for the helicopter after he arrived just by chance on the scene. We were so grateful that Rachel, the hospital chaplain who had helped us so much in December, could join us as well. She later told me what amazement she felt being able to watch the four of us as a family, interacting and being together just like we should be; she of all people knew how miraculous it was to have regained part of our lives that was supposed to have been gone forever. It was so apparent in everyone's faces they couldn't believe how great Brian was doing and how happy they were to see and meet him in these better circumstances.

Dr. Braz was hoping that both boys could come up on stage at the end of the concert to assist him with a special song he planned to play, and in deciding we could do this, Brian also said he wanted to talk while he was onstage. We thought it would be very touching if Brian thanked the crowd for being there, so we began to try to prepare what he could say. Ben (as usual the jokester) said, "You should get up there and say, 'I'm Brian, and I like Statesboro and PIE!' and everyone will laugh." In the head of a brain-injured child, certain phrases or jokes can sometimes get stuck on rewind (a trait the psychologists called perseveration). Before long, Brian had morphed our suggestion and Ben's into a statement he kept saying over and over. By the time the moment came when he actually got up to the microphone, he really did say, "Thank you for the prayers Statesboro. I like Statesboro . . . and pie . . . but mostly pie." Getting a roar of applause and cheers only helped cement this phrase into Brian's repertoire, and he would say this to us many times after this (hoping for that positive feedback again I'm sure!).

Brian had always had a strong musical side; we would hear him singing at church for example, perfectly on pitch. But if we made mention of it, he would immediately stop in a reflex of stubbornness. But throughout his recovery, it was clear that playing music made a huge difference for his recovery. One way that we entertained him as he began to regain his ability to stand and walk was to play a dance videogame. The idea is to mimic the dance moves that are on the screen, and he did just okay with that part (given he had barely regained his strength and balance, this was not surprising). But he very loudly sang along with the pop songs that were part of the game. I guess his reticence to sing aloud went when the frontal lobe, which controls inhibition, was damaged. He sometimes wanted to turn it on just to hear the music. He also loved going to bed each night with his Kidz Bop CDs, and knew every song by heart.

A popular song during this time was Katy Perry's "Firework." The song's message is about hanging on and not giving in, because someday your circumstances can turn from a struggle to a celebration. A friend wrote me one day and said that her son (who was about the same age as Brian) told her that every time he heard that song, he just thought about Brian. He told his mom, "Brian really is like fireworks. He's just going to keep on showing everybody." For another child to recognize this was true to Brian's life was really touching to me. It became a song that always gave me hope when I heard it. But it was almost enough to give me goose bumps when we were able to walk with Brian into his classroom after being away from school for nine months, and heard what song playing on the loudspeaker ... yes, "Firework." It was just a little reminder from God that he's always giving us signs. For us, music has been a saving, healing, and necessary part of Brian's recovery, and important for the whole family as well.

16

Brothers (Sibling Therapy)

Ben and his little brother have always had an interesting sibling relationship. Their personalities are so different from each other; it could have led them to not get along at all. They are almost exactly three years and six months apart in age—a gap that could in some cases lead to a pretty big separation. Those details have made some impact on them through the years, but all in all, I have always been impressed by the loyalty, love, and interest they've shown in each other.

When I was pregnant with Brian and Ben was only three years old, we began to toss around baby names. David and I both had some favorites, but nothing was coming up as a clear winner. So one day while driving, we started asking Ben. "Is the baby's name Kevin?" "Is the baby's name Alex?" "Is the baby's name David?" Each name got a firm resounding "No!" from Ben. We pretty much assumed he was playing a game of having fun saying no to everything we asked until we said, "Is the baby's name Brian?" Ben looked right at us and said, "Uh . . . yeah!" (teenage-like "no-duh" implied). I always felt like he was thinking, "What took you guys so

0

long to figure *that* out?" David and I looked at each other, gave a head nod to say, "I'm good with that," and it was decided.

It had been my intention to *not* name our second child with the same initial as our first, though I know many families like that tradition. If anything, knowing that we would have two "B" names almost did in the name Brian for me. But somehow, when Ben was so certain of it, I just felt he was right. I came to completely and totally love the name, and have always felt it suited Brian. A typical boy—athletic, active, rather stoic and quiet at times yet friendly and quick to laugh when amused. A name that stands the test of your lifetime . . . you can imagine a Brian being four or twenty-four or seventy-four. It was just one of the first of many times that Ben's influence played a huge role when it came to his brother.

After the accident, as Ben recovered from his injuries, he would have had every right to be jealous of the time that David and I were spending in Brian's room. Yes, he had our family and friends with him nearly twenty-four-seven, but he went through a pretty terrible ordeal as well. Who wouldn't want their mom and dad with them after that? Being able to sneak away for a couple of hours with Ben during those first few days was such a relief. I cherished being able to talk to him, give him hugs, and to be so grateful he was recovering fairly quickly. I have never seen such a young kid be so generous with his heart as Ben when he implicitly gave us permission to let our loved ones take over for us and be his primary companions during those days. He never complained, he always wanted for us to tell him how his brother was doing, and when gifts and presents came, he pointed out which ones were going to be for Brian once he got better.

As the day came that we had to tell Ben that the doctors had not given Brian any hope for recovering, and that we thought he would be going up to heaven, it fell on David to break the news. The first thing Ben wanted to know was "Can't the doctors be wrong?" He was determined to not give up at any point on his little brother. The child-life specialist helped Ben make a handprint artwork that had both he and Brian's hands, then spent some time with him and us trying to help make the transition easier. The love Ben had for Brian was just so strong and plain to see. He didn't get hysterical, though of course we were all crying, and he talked to Brian and said good-bye to him when it was time to go. I think I know now that somehow Ben's soul was tuned in to what God intended for Brian though, because that good-bye was "I'll see you later" even though none of us thought Ben would ever see Brian alive again.

As it turns out, Ben was the one who had been right all along. When the situation turned, and we brought Brian to the Ogeechee Area Hospice in Statesboro two days after Ben had said good-bye to him, Ben did see his brother again. I still do not recall that Ben ever reacted in a way that showed he thought Brian was actually about to die though. It is my hunch that Ben's soul just got that message from God that the rest of us were too overcome with worry to hear.

As the days at the hospice went on and on, we were drawing closer and closer to Christmas. Not that we had any energy or time to be Christmas shopping, but our friends finally gently encouraged us to spend an hour one day arranging presents for Ben. I can remember being so stressed and worried about being away from the hospice during that time. But obviously, Ben deserved for his parents to get him Christmas presents. What I never expected was that around that same time, Ben himself asked me, "Mom, aren't we going to go buy some Christmas presents for Brian?" My heart was so nearly broken at this point. Ben still believed Brian could wake up, could live, and would want to have Christmas presents. In the state of shock we had been living in, we were still expecting it would be any moment that God would take Brian, so we hadn't planned to buy him presents. To Ben, it only made sense that we *would* buy Brian presents.

Ben's aunt took him to the bookstore in town, and they picked out a stuffed toy from a collection called the Ugly Doll Citizens. It was a pretty typical little boy decision, since the dolls were intentionally designed to not be too cutesy but to have funny, weird or strange-looking appearances. The doll he picked out for Brian was named Nopy. Many things took on an added level of poignancy in our lives at this point, and it was really a moment of inspiration when Ben gave Brian his present on Christmas Eve. Over the course of the last few days leading up to Christmas, inspired by Ben's faith, we had decided to follow Ben's lead and believe that Brian may be able to survive. The message found on the nametag of the doll gave us goose bumps, and really seemed too amazing to be a coincidence.

Nopy is small.
Nopy is a wee lad.
Nopy is HUGE!
That's right!
He may be small on the outside, but has big dreams,
big ideas, and a big plan for the two of you.
You're into being a part of something big, right?
Follow little Nopy.
He'll make it happen for you.
Big time!

Were we into being part of something big? We had no idea how spot-on that description would be. And just like Nopy, even though Brian himself was a small boy, the power of the miracle in his life is *huge*! Yet again, we looked at Ben in amazement when without even trying he got it exactly right.

During Brian's hospitalization at the rehabilitation unit (CIRU), Ben was able to come and visit him on the weekends, and usually one to two other evenings a week after school. I can remember so vividly bringing in a dinner (usually supplied by one of the many generous neighbors who took turns cooking for us) and the four of us would have dinner together in a small break room just outside of the CIRU. Brian was in his wheelchair, the rest of us crowded around a small table. Ben would talk to Brian, telling him about his day, the stuff that was going on in fifth grade, and even though Brian still couldn't speak at this point, you could see he was listening to his big brother. One day the head of Rehabilitation Services at the hospital (who was one of the physicians on rounds) asked about

Brian's brother. I can remember so clearly his advice to me. "Have his brother around him as much as possible. One of the best things I can recommend for him is 'sibling therapy.' We see it all the time." We took this to heart, and tried to be sure that only one or two days went by without Ben visiting. Finally, we were given our discharge date—February 7. We were both happy and terrified, because Brian was still so debilitated at that point. He still couldn't speak, sit up, eat, or drink, and was getting lots of medications throughout the day. How would we handle this?

The day came when Ben and Brian were finally under the same roof again. It had been over two months since Ben had his little brother at home, and the photos we took that first night were all of Ben and Brian together. No, they didn't look anything like the ones we had taken just a couple of months before. But they were both smiling and they were together. And at that moment, that was enough, and we were so grateful.

And then, the best part of all. Just as the doctor predicted, having Ben around more of the time seemed to accelerate Brian's recovery. Though he still was far from being able to eat, during meals we would wheel Brian up to the table across from Ben, and we would try to do what we had always done. One day at the table, Ben asked Brian something, and he was sure that Brian answered him. I, not having heard it, was skeptical. But later that day, it happened again. Before long, we had deciphered a list of twenty or so words that we had heard Brian say. Ben took credit for hearing the first words that Brian said, and we were just so happy to hear him talking again.

The speech was slurred and without much breath support, so it sounded more like a whisper. His mouth was still distorted from the accident, and he had to work on closing it completely when trying to make sounds. But it was amazing how fast we went from having him totally uncommunicative, to him attempting some unclear head nodding, to him actually speaking again. It was only after he was around his brother every day that this occurred, so, Ben, I do give you credit.

Another milestone came a few weeks after being home. Brian was to practice eating, but the food had to be extremely soft. Since baby food was not something he enjoyed the taste of, I had started buying pudding cups with soft peaches (the package called it a peach parfait, which sounds pretty gourmet, but really, it was pudding with fruit). For some reason one day, Ben started to call this "peach poop." If you do not have elementary school boys, I will stop for a moment to say that anything and everything related to poop, farts, boogers, or any other bodily function is not just funny to them, it's hilarious! As Ben teased his brother saying, "Aren't you going to eat your peach poop?" we finally heard a beautiful sound we'd been missing all those months—Brian laughing.

When you stop and think about it, a laugh is a universal sound that makes us happy just hearing it. You could hear someone laughing who spoke any language, from any culture, and you would understand that person was feeling happiness, joy, and amusement at that moment. It is a beautiful thing to hear, especially when it had been taken away from our son for so long. He certainly hadn't had much to laugh about during the weeks he lived in a hospital. And you could argue the severely damaged state he was still in at that time didn't give much to laugh about either, but the beauty of two brothers just laughing over a poop joke overpowered all of that.

We came to depend on Ben's influence in helping encourage Brian in so many facets of his recovery. I feel certain that wanting to please his brother was as strong a motivator for Brian as anything. From Ben's end, every time he helped get Brian to do something that helped him get better, the closer he was to having his little brother back the way he had been before. Still, I sometimes struggled with putting too much of a burden on Ben. After all, as a ten-year-old boy it shouldn't be your job to help someone recover from a life-threatening injury. In the end though, I believe it was the most natural thing our family could have done; coming together to find what would work, each of us, even Ben, playing our own part.

As Brian's recovery moved forward and he gained back some of the physical skills that he had lost, his emotional recovery became more difficult. In a way, the early months of the recovery were the most difficult for us, but perhaps easier for Brian, in that he was not really able to process the scope of the changes that had occurred to him. Once he reached higher levels of awareness, he justifiably began acting out and having real moments of anger and frustration. This was an extremely difficult phase for me personally to deal with, and thankfully, I had professional help that aided my own understanding of the process as a whole. Ben was quick to step in when Brian would get into one of these moods, and would do something silly or distracting in order to snap Brian out of the tantrum.

What I appreciate so much about Ben doing this was the intuitive way he knew just what to say and usually also when to say it. Sometimes Ben did become frustrated and angry with Brian for the behavior Brian was exhibiting towards David or me, but more often, he rather calmly saw the opportunity to play a part in diffusing the situation in a way that only he could. The responsibility he took on himself was a very mature and loving component. Don't get me wrong, he was still a kid. He still got annoyed or frustrated himself when he had to be told "no" or when we had to tend to something for Brian rather than him. But in all, Ben's ability to be a happy, typical fifth- or sixth-grade kid while his family went through this ordeal has been amazing.

It is a mystery why this miracle happened, but I do ponder whether it has really been for Ben's sake that it did. One day we may know for sure, but in the meantime, I am thankful every day that both of my boys get to grow up with each other.

17

Return to School

Brian was born in October, ensuring that he was always one of the oldest kids in his class in school. The year of the accident as a first grader, he had already turned seven, and these extra few months of life compared to younger kids gave him a real advantage academically. He was excelling in school, loved the order of the classroom, was particularly excited about math, and just generally was a good student. The Thanksgiving of 2011, one week before the accident, Brian read a whole chapter book for the first time, and was so proud that he'd done something just like his big brother. And of course, we were proud of him too.

How difficult it was a couple of short months later as he began to return to us to see how debilitated he was. It was almost impossible to imagine the boy we saw in the early stages of his recovery back in a classroom. However, the signs were there that Brian could indeed meet that challenge. As early as February, when Brian began to speak again, we would write words on a whiteboard or paper and he would read the words to us. After hearing so many worst-case scenarios and not having seen any real evidence ourselves by that point that he would regain his cognitive skills, it was an amazing thing to see. We began to put small math problems down, or simply ask him questions like, "What is ten plus seven," and sure enough, he would answer in a whisper, "Seventeen." We began to consider that he really was still okay from that perspective, deep inside, even if his communication skills were still limited.

Around the time he started the Day Rehabilitation program in late March of that spring, the social worker there encouraged us to begin the process of re-enrolling him in our local school system. In order to be considered for special education and services, he would need to be a currently enrolled student, whether he was actually able to attend or not. However, one option she also told us to ask about was home-based teaching. In that program, students who had medical issues that prevented them from attending school could have a teacher assigned to come to their hospital room or home in order to try to keep up with their work. There was a teacher at the Day Rehabilitation facility, but unfortunately, because that was located in a different county than ours, Brian would not be able to utilize that teacher officially during his time. Once this became clear, we immediately made the request from our elementary school to find a teacher to work with Brian.

Ms. Terry Johnson was a kindergarten teacher at the school, and happened to be a neighbor, living just a few blocks away. She was assigned to provide about three hours a week of teaching time to Brian. At the time, he was riding a bus provided by CHOA to the Day Rehab location (about six miles away) and arrived back home each day around four p.m. (A reality of Atlanta traffic is that no one finds this abnormal at all, six miles taking sixty minutes.) To say Brian had been through a lot by this point each day was an understatement. Yet, three days a week, upon arriving home, Brian and Ms. Johnson would work on material appropriate for his grade and his abilities.

He could barely hold anything, much less write coherently, but they worked on identifying letters, numbers, and shapes. I remember her surprise one day when she brought in a new set of flash cards with three-dimensional shapes, and Brian was able to name most of them. He named a pyramid, a cylinder, a cube, and so on. She looked at him with such surprise, because those words and concepts seemed so advanced. But it was just another sign that Brian's intelligence and competitive spirit were alive and well.

As the school year ended, so did Ms. Johnson's contract. Brian continued at Day Rehab for another few weeks into the summer, and as he prepared to discharge, his speech therapists (who also do cognitive work with patients) reported he was beginning to complete assignments in basic math, reading, comprehension, and spelling. While his shortened attention span and impulsive lack of self-control were still strongly affecting his ability to do the work, it was not the difficulty of the work itself that was a problem. As we made arrangements for him to return to school in August, another psychological test was performed.

The psychologists had some very systematic and complex assessments that they gave Brian in order to assess his levels of preparedness for the school setting. In Brian's case, he tired and bored easily and at several points simply refused to complete portions of the exam. Even still, Brian was scoring in normal ranges for many of their criteria. Some areas were certainly below average, but even the psychologists recognized their results would have likely been much higher had his attention issues not prevented him from completing the test. In any case, we were not as concerned with these results as we were with providing it to the school district in order to start the process of creating an Individual Education Plan (IEP) for Brian once the school year started.

Amazingly, Brian was able to enroll as a second grader in August of that year back at our local elementary school. For a short period of time earlier in the summer (when Brian was still utilizing a wheelchair), some staff had suggested he may need to attend another elementary school in the county, which had additional services for physically disabled kids. We were just so convinced he would thrive by being back at his former school, back with his friends and familiar teachers, that we hoped he would not be sent to a different location. Our fears were relieved when we finally met with the special education coordinator a few weeks before school started, and she agreed he could re-enroll at Evansdale Elementary, and would be set up to receive services.

As in most schools these days, special education students are now incorporated into the general classroom as much of the time as possible. For Brian, this meant he had a homeroom second grade teacher and was part of that class, but did leave for a special classroom with more one-on-one instruction for his core subject areas of language arts and math. This arrangement was a good compromise, because Brian was able to get out of the larger classroom about half of the day, and yet, had an identity as part of that homeroom class (something that is important to elementary school kids).

Brian also had the assistance of a paraprofessional Ms. Middlebrook. She is truly an angel on earth, and much like some of his other therapists and helpers, she came to love and appreciate Brian for all of his wonderful, loving, and funny characteristics. All the while, she was usually taking the brunt of the poor behavior choices that he might make on any given day. Never taking anything personally, she just quietly and firmly provided him help as he needed it. At first, it was supervision when walking in the halls and going to the restroom, helping him carry his tray or getting his lunch ready, and providing extra help during class for him to stay on track and follow instructions. As the year went on, those physical limitations lessened, and he continued to return slowly but surely to being more independent at school. So much of that independence was thanks to her!

Generally, he was excited to be back at school so things started out going fine. It didn't take too long into the year, however, before the strain of all that had changed in his world began to take a toll on him. As Brian gained more awareness of his own differences and deficiencies, he began to act out with inappropriate and even defiant behavior. While not unexpected in someone with as severe an injury in the frontal lobe of the brain (where impulse control is found), if Brian became upset about something, he had no inhibition in showing his feelings. Many kids struggle with behavior issues in school, but it was just very difficult to see Brian having these because he had always been such a model student before.

Adjustments were made, including allowing Brian more time with the resource teacher rather than the large class, and a behavior chart was created with the help of the speech therapist to provide him a way to get positive rewards for staying on track each period of the day. We also began bringing Brian to a child psychologist that fall to help him with dealing with the anger, frustration, and irritation that was coming from this dramatic change in his life.

The year continued, and with further adjustments in medications and just his generally improving health all around, he did manage to function in the school environment. Again, it was not the same as he had been before, but his academic grades were still good, and he and his dad even began the challenge of completing reading assignments then testing them in the Accelerated Reading program (AR). Though all students participated in AR, it probably wouldn't have mattered much if Brian's level had been fairly low. However, Brian (with David's help) not only met his grade level point goal, he surpassed it by the end of second grade. It was just another example that never giving up on the goal would pay off in the end.

As awards day came around in late May of that year, we proudly watched as Brian walked up the steps of the stage, walked across when his name was called, shook hands with the principal, and received his awards for reading and general academic recognition. Who could have imagined the little boy we first heard reading us a few short words could take on this challenge and be this successful? The challenges will remain for Brian in this arena for many years to come in some form or fashion, but we are confident that each year he will just continue to progress further and further. It will not surprise me at all when he finishes high school, college, or even graduate school one day.

Months later, as Brian's awareness of the events that occurred improved, he made a surprising and poignant comment. I was helping him complete a portion of a science project during his third grade year and said to him, "Good job, Brian, you have a smart brain." He turned to me, patted himself on the head a few times, and said, "Me and this old thing have been through a lot together."

I laughed, but when I remembered how far Brian had come from the days when doctors thought he might never communicate at all, it really hit home. During his stay in the rehabilitation hospital, his sole mode of communication was non-verbal head movements, and eventually, the use of a button that he could use to answer "yes" to questions we asked. For some TBI patients, that might be the only way they could ever again communicate with the rest of the world. But not Brian! Hearing him make jokes and show an intellect that can incorporate humor about his own difficult journey is just an example of a long string of accomplishments he has made in his cognitive recovery. It shows me that his intelligence, while impaired by impulses and attention difficulties now, is still strong, and gives me complete hope for the future.

Part Three:

Lessons in Faith

I have no theological background, but I am a person of faith. By writing this book, I am trying to follow what I believe is God's plan for me, namely to give others hope by sharing the extraordinary events of Brian's miraculous recovery. It would be a somewhat safer venture if I were to stop at this point to just let the events themselves be the story. Yet, I have heard a voice in my head saying to write on. The following short essays are reflections on my journey through this experience from a faith-based perspective, and I humbly offer them up, flawed and imperfect as they are, from my heart and as honestly relayed as I can.

18

Faith in the Unknown

I write about my faith in this book because there is no way to write this book and *not* talk about faith. But over the course of Brian's recovery, I think one of the most surprising things has been my need to share my insights related to what God's part of this miracle has been, and what impacts it has had on the way I think, feel, and view the world around me. It's been a piece of my identity that I have held guarded and close to me my entire life—originally out of fear of rejection, later a sort of laissez-fare attitude of "I'm going to worry about my spiritual life, it's not my job to affect others." And even now, it's somewhat scary to lay this piece of my experience out for the world to see and to judge.

I have learned to appreciate the strength that comes from having others pray for me. During some of the darkest moments of this time, if I wrote on our blog asking for prayers the response came thundering back more than I could have imagined. It was not long before I felt compelled to simply write what I felt, without regard to who would read it, even if I would have never in a million years said some of the things I could write aloud to others. I feel God's work in me in my ability to be more open in sharing my beliefs and insights. After all, we all go through trials and frustrations in life, but don't we all want to know that they can be overcome?

During Brian's initial two weeks in the Pediatric ICU, there was not a day that I didn't spend in prayer. I remember despite the numbness and overwhelming pain of seeing our baby in such terrible shape that a calm and sense of peace could be found as I sat by his bedside and prayed. I was praying the rosary as each day ended and most of the commotion had quieted. The rosary is misunderstood by some, but to me, it is a beautiful connection to God. Each night I prayed for the blessed mother to intervene for Brian. It was a meditation, a plea for help, and a centering force for me, all wrapped up in one. I simply prayed, from one mother to another, that she would understand this heartache and petition to God on our behalf. I felt a sense of peace and love each time I finished, and it was always the last thing that I did before I left his side to get a few hours of sleep each evening.

Brian's room was the closest to the nurses' station, as he was very clearly the sickest patient they had at that time. The sounds of the monitors beeping, the telephone ringing, the nurses and doctors relaying orders were virtually nonstop. Yet, there was a feeling expressed by many visitors to Brian's room that they just felt an overwhelming sense of God's presence when they walked across the threshold. What physical effect does prayer have in our three-dimensional world? Can it impact the air around us? It felt that way in Brian's room. I believe that God had sent a spirit (guardian angel, a departed family member, or The Holy Spirit himself) to be with Brian and this is what was being felt by those attuned to sensing it. Another person compared it to the sense of peace and tranquility she always felt when she was visiting a convent where the nuns spent hours each day in prayer and meditation. This physical sensation was shared by those in Brian's presence both in Savannah and after we arrived in Atlanta. It is a mystery and we will never know for certain, but I am so comforted in thinking back and imagining every molecule in that space just filled up with the light and energy of God.

Throughout this time, I prayed for Brian to recover. I prayed for strength to handle this situation. I prayed for Ben, and asked God to help him even while we couldn't. I know that while I wanted to believe God was in control of the situation, I still feared the worst. I had every rational reason to believe the doctors' predictions that Brian was gone to us already, whether he was still breathing or not. I did not pray for a miracle for Brian while we were at the PICU. I prayed for strength to accept God's will for Brian. I prayed this because I thought it was the right thing to do. We say in the Lord's Prayer "Thy will be done" every time we pray it, but it is so hard to really mean that we can trust that God's plan is the best. Don't we all as human beings want to pretend we know the best way for ourselves, our kids, our friends, our adversaries? We are conditioned to try to find solutions and answers; allowing God to control the situation just goes against all we're used to. And so, I thought by praying that I could accept God's will, I was getting closer to the path he wanted me to follow.

As we made the incredibly difficult and heartbreaking decision to remove Brian from the ventilator, we thought we were surrendering our child to God himself. There is a peace that came from the sense that in heaven Brian would have no pain or sadness, and that we could take on that burden if this was the way God wanted it to be. The ventilator removed, it was the worst type of anticipation that followed, thinking it was going to be any minute, any second, and our beautiful boy would take his last breath. As I have already written, God not only provided the answer, he provided us the inspiration to finally ask the hardest question we could ask: God, will you please give us a miracle? And in his glorious love for us, he did just that.

It was in many ways because of this strong belief that I had in God's clear answer to my prayer that I could endure the uncertainty and pain of the following weeks. In the world of rehabilitation (and maybe medicine more generally), it is pretty common for the patient to be given a "worst-case" scenario. One friend of David's, who is a nurse, described it like reading the entire warning label of a bottle of Tylenol. If you ever read the potential side effects for some of the most common medicines we use, you might never use them. The doctors were giving us the "warning label" in a way, and I guess they would rather be wrong and have the recovery be better than expected than the other way around. It is also the case that in TBI patients so much is unknown about how the brain recovers, and what an ultimate outcome will be for an individual. So, while it was painful and stressful at the time to hear these dire predictions, I felt like the knowledge I held in my heart (that God provided us this miracle after we asked) was stronger than the terrible predicted outcomes. It's a metaphor used so often in spiritual writings, but it felt like God had anchored me, given me a rock to rest on, and from that place of solid love, I could move through the day-to-day process.

Sometimes it almost felt like I had a secret that none of the therapists knew; they saw the state Brian was in, and very logically determined only an extremely limited recovery was likely. I looked at where we had been and *knew* in my heart that it was happening in God's time, and he was going to bring Brian back to us.

In revisiting our journals on our blog, it is both heartbreaking and heartwarming to go back and see how this faith played out during the first few weeks back in Atlanta. We rejoiced and celebrated the progress Brian made, no matter how tiny. We marveled when he began to make sounds (not speak, mind you, just moan) because we hadn't heard a sound from his mouth in weeks. We were in awe and appreciation of the many kind gifts of food and care that our neighbors and friends provided, for the visits, for the prayers from so many friends and strangers alike. It's almost like two opposing forces going on to describe what it was like to interact with Brian during those weeks—wanting to feel optimistic and have faith, but having the reality that your child can only moan and not speak pulling you toward despair. God gave me so much strength during this time; I have no explanation for how I managed to get up day after day and be pulled toward the fear and the despair and yet not let it overtake me.

I wrote on a particularly difficult day the following passage:

Imagine if you woke up every morning and the only and first thing you think about is your child having to go through this. There is no escape, even in the twilight hour when you should be coming out of a restful sleep and ready to hit the day. I have to fight against the temptation to give in to the despair of it all. It is so hard to fight that! Many of you have told me privately it's okay to write about the hard times, yet David and I tend to stay away from writing about that.

Part of it is to remind myself that going down that self-pity pathway just doesn't help anything. Don't get me wrong, plenty of days I can brush those worries aside quickly and get on with it. Other days (like yesterday), they just linger. In particular yesterday, a couple of small issues here (that have been resolved, thank goodness) got me annoyed and then that annoyance turns into "If I weren't here in the first place, I wouldn't even have to deal with this."

I'm definitely guilty of being "instant gratification oriented" just like the rest of the US population. You know, if you want to know just Google it. If you want to eat—the pre-prepared frozen meal or just fast food. So this is smacking me in the face with a huge dose of "You just have to wait to see what will happen to Brian, and oh, by the way, we can't tell you how long you'll have to wait." It's a special challenge to keep the motivation going with no end in sight. It's kind of interesting, because of course even they realize this here and talk to me for example, when they are stretching Brian's muscles or doing something uncomfortable or painful they always will tell him, "We'll do this for a count of ten" because it's just too hard if he has to endure something painful and has no idea when it will end.

Indeed . . .

It has been a blessing to me personally to realize a deeper level of faith in God during this time. I appreciate so much that ability to connect in ways I never had before, and it provides a sense of reassurance and peace to everything in my life. The hope of this book has always been to share some of this understanding with those who don't have a crisis or tragedy of their own, but who may find their own challenges or trials in life to be easier to manage once viewed from the perspectives shared here.

19

Perseverance

Perseverance can be seen as a series of actions, but to me, more accurately, perseverance is a mindset. The mental determination required to carry out the work at hand regardless of the difficulties. If not for perseverance, none of Brian's amazing rehabilitation would have been possible; I do know this for sure.

Yes, I could (and did) write about the tedium of the actions we repeated day after day after day during Brian's recovery. Many of these actions occur still to this day, and honestly, may forever. The severity of the repercussions of *not* completing some of these actions has lessened, but that does not take away from the fact that they continue to exist. We went from grinding and administering medicines to Brian through his g-tube on a complex schedule through the day and night to eventually giving him about four pills in a day—one at breakfast and lunch and two at night. Back then, the stakes were so high, and no matter how tedious and tiring it was, we never faltered, never failed to give him exactly what he was prescribed at exactly the right hour.

His schedule of outpatient therapies has drawn down considerably, but they still exist. I am sure to pick him up from school on time, have snacks and a drink in the car, and off we go to one of a few locations in the Atlanta area for rehabilitation sessions two to three times a week. It's a pattern of actions that at one time were incredibly difficult to pull off, especially when he was wheelchair bound and I was alone trying to transport him to these offices. Now, though Brian walks to the car, puts himself inside, buckles his own seatbelt, and holds his own snack while we drive, it's still an act of perseverance to continue to do this week after week. I am so grateful for the people he sees who have helped him to progress, yet honestly, it was often a tiring and defeating process.

There is no way around it; in our human condition, we are so quick to forget the benefit of the big picture when we're working toward our goals. Trying to lose weight? We all know, eat fewer calories, exercise more, and make smart choices. But in the moment, the chips just look so good. The donut is tempting you. We completely choose to forget the goal in those moments, instead of persevering with the harder path, we cave in. I am just like anyone else when it comes to these weaknesses. And that is why I am writing this chapter, because I know this truth applies to all of us.

Through a gift from God, I was given the strength to persevere through this accident. I always admired people who had stories of terrible things happening to them, and then they turned those things around into something positive. But I never saw myself in that light, until now. I would have never predicted I had the internal strength to make it through some of the things that I have had to do. And yet, here I am. I have never been more confident in my life that I was aided and guided so that this story would have the conclusion that it does. I include our whole family as having received this blessing actually, because David and Ben have endured many of these very same trials and have never stopped being willing to keep going.

When we asked God for a true miracle that night in the hospice, the answer that flooded through my mind the next day was that our job was to do the work. God's job was to change whatever needed to change in Brian's physical body in order for him to have the capacity to recover. Our work was (and still is) to recognize this miracle, and to persevere through *whatever* came in order to fulfill it.

It occurred to me that this is like life itself. How we come to be living in this world is a miracle in its own right. God saw to it that our physical bodies and our souls exist. Miraculous! Now, it is up to us to do the work in order for these lives to have meaning. We cannot do it without God, but he relies on us to do our part, to do the work. In third grade, Brian was given a homework assignment to write a paragraph to answer this prompt: Write about a time you showed perseverance.

 I remember one time when I showed perseverance when I worked at getting stronger. Sometimes I didn't want to but I kept on going. When I was standing in the stander, and I didn't want to but I did. I kept on doing it, until Dad took it back to the company with Adam. It made me feel pretty good because I was standing on the floor on my feet. And I couldn't eat when I had the feeding tube, but I went with it until the day they got rid of it (and I got a second belly button!) And when they took it out I was afraid it was going to hurt, but it didn't hurt at all. When I think about these things I think I'm pretty strong.

We are all equipped more than we know to persevere through any difficulty that this life may send our way. In a beautiful way, keeping the mindset of dedication and belief in the goal is honoring God's plan for us, and in the end, really the only way we can do it. One step, one hour, one day at a time.

20

Community

Leaving our small college town of Statesboro in the summer of 2011 was particularly difficult for me. Living there, for the first time in my adult life, I felt part of a community. I was surrounded by colleagues in my work environment both on campus and across the region through my professional organization that I valued and enjoyed. I felt a strong connection to our church, was able to take a leadership role in the music ministry there, and felt happy just to be a part of a strong faith community. But most of all, I had made the best friends in that small town.

A fairly small community, many people associated with the university (like we were) got to know each other quite easily. It was a quick process to form and then reinforce friendships when you literally might see someone in several different environments—at the downtown festival, out at the little league park, at work, at church, surely if nothing else, at the grocery store. Though a small place, there were so many social activities going on all the time, and we very quickly were not just immersed in them, we were making really close friends.

Atlanta—that was a different story. Though plenty of great people live in a city of this size, there is no way to replicate the convenience of having the same people show up in different spheres of your life. The people you worked with were not the people in your kids' school, and the people in the neighborhood may never go to the same events or festivals you did, and so on. Initially, I was really struggling with the loss of having our close friends, and can remember praying to God during those first couple of months in our new home, "Please, send me friends." They say prayers are always answered, just not in the way you sometimes expect. God certainly sent me friends. But first came the most devastating event of my life.

I have already described the selfless and unbelievable dedication that these same Statesboro friends showed to us during not only our first month following the accident, but even when we returned home to Atlanta. I can never repay them, and I will be grateful for them my whole life. But it is a different group of "friends" that I think is the surprising piece of this answered prayer.

As I wrote earlier, the power of this story was compelling to people. The online journal on our CaringBridge page and our Facebook prayer group page became the way in which God brought us thousands of "friends" just when we needed it most. It is fairly common to see people forward requests for prayers the way that originally others did for our family, but I have rarely seen the word spread in quite the way it did in our family's case. So many times, as we posted our specific prayer requests, we saw real results in some kind of physical or psychological way.

I imagine it something like this: through this experience, though I might have wanted to stay positive and close to God, it was like I was floating on a big sea of depression, anxiety, and even despair. It would have been so easy to just slowly slip into that sea, and let it overtake me. It was always there, always calling for me. What kept that from happening was a virtual wall of prayer coming from these thousands of people, most of whom we had never met nor would ever meet. It was like they were lifting me up to God, as if I was secure on top of their upstretched hands in that sea of fear. Sure, I knew it was down there, but I never slipped in.

The love and devotion shown by so many families, in particular by the children who prayed for Brian and Ben every night, was just the most beautiful thing to witness. The gifts of food, cards, books, blankets, toys, etc. are too numerous to even begin to detail. The acts of kindness on a larger scale were given to us as well, like David's college friends building a ramp for our house or Dr. Braz staging a concert for our benefit. We can only hope to pay forward these generous gifts and try to do our best to adequately thank those who gave them. It was so amazing to have been shown such love.

As the prayer map that recorded locations of prayers from all around the world showed me, my community of support was literally everywhere. Even in Fiji, where someone simply agreed to say a prayer when the story was told, and yet, in that small action showed me that we are truly all connected. We are all a community. And I have no reason to fear that I don't have friends; God sent me more than I could have ever imagined.

21

Forgiveness

Once people have gotten to know me enough that they are comfortable asking, I very often am questioned about how my father-in-law is doing. It's usually with a grave, somewhat hesitant expression. They wonder how it is that he is dealing with this accident, since he was the driver. Though never spoken directly, I also understand people's curiosity and concern about how we are doing with him. In other words, "Have we forgiven him?"

The second most common question I have been asked in this regard involves the staff at the Memorial Hospital in Savannah. Because 100 percent of the therapists, social workers, doctors, and nurses who have treated Brian since we returned to Atlanta saw him only "post-miracle" as I would call it, they are typically shocked to learn he had ever been sent to hospice care. "Don't you just want to go back to that hospital and tell them off?" is the basic gist of what I have been asked on many occasions.

Here's the truth: in both cases, there is zero animosity, zero bitterness, and zero anger. In a completely real way, God performed another miracle in this family that is just as awe-inspiring as helping Brian survive. He helped my heart spontaneously forgive.

This shocks me in many ways, because though in life I find myself to be very loyal and dedicated to the people I love, I also acknowledge the darker side of that loyalty. If you betray my trust, I can cut you out of my life without a second thought. It's not always experiences of a totally serious nature. Bad service at a restaurant causes my parents to miss a plane? I won't return to that restaurant (or any of that chain) for years. Bad experience with a place of work? I would go out of my way not to know anything about former colleagues or supervisors, despite us having mutual friends. Some issues were more serious. Mistreated in high school? I was happy to leave not only my hometown, but my home state and have never considered returning to live. It's not something I am proud of; it's a reactionary trait I am sure came about as a way to defend myself from being hurt.

So, you can see why it would be understandable that I might bear some ill will for the events of December 2011. Probably no one would blame me if, because of the pain we went through, I just couldn't bear to have a relationship with my father-in-law again. Most might think it is totally justified if I were to want nothing to do with Memorial Hospital, or anyone who worked there. After all, my precious baby was nearly taken from me, and even when his life was spared, the aftermath that we have all lived through has been far from easy.

In my spiritual life, studying forgiveness has been an important element that helped me gain an appreciation for the level of love God has for us. Our former pastor, Father Tim McKeown, used to preach from spiritual readings he had done of the images of God forgiving us. He would say that if God were the ocean, when we ask for forgiveness it's like we are throwing a handful of sand (our sins) into the giant, rolling waves. We may have two handfuls, a bucket, we could even have a huge dumpster full of sand. Once we toss it on the ocean (God) it's dispersed, gone, never could we return those individual grains of sand together again. That's how strong God's love is, and that's what forgiveness looks like.

How difficult it is for us humans to practice anything close to this level of forgiveness though. Our own egos, fears, pride, they all get in the way, and make us think that holding on to some kind of anger or resentment is the solution. My faith teaches me if I wish to be forgiven, I must forgive. And though I may know in my mind this is the way, my heart still fails to live up to this standard on so many occasions.

Yet, when I first laid my eyes on my father-in-law after the accident, my heart was completely flooded with concern, love, and forgiveness. It wasn't even a conscious thought, like "I am going to forgive him." It was just already present in my heart from the first moment. Any of us could have been in his shoes, but more than that, he obviously loves Brian and Ben so much and would never harm them intentionally. How much more difficult would this recovery have been if my heart had been too blinded with anger or bitterness to focus on what was really important—helping Brian get better?

As I described earlier, returning Brian to the care of the physicians at Memorial who had given us the prognosis that he wouldn't live wasn't difficult for me. I did *not* want to find them and curse them out. I only wanted to show them Brian and what a change had occurred in him. I do not guess that pediatric neurosurgeons or trauma doctors have the luxury to get emotionally involved in their patients' lives. But I do know that it's a significant statement when a doctor in that environment would say to me, "There are some things that medicine just cannot explain."

How did my positive and forgiving attitude toward those doctors influence not only their perception of Brian's recovery, but how they may treat other patients going forward? I do not blame them for making the "wrong" diagnosis, because I honestly do not believe they did. I believe fully that God *can* and *did* make physical changes in Brian's brain that altered our future. Doctors cannot predict when and if God would do such a miracle, so how could I hold any resentment toward them for doing what they were trained to do—tell us what they saw at that time from a scientific perspective.

I know the battle in the human heart between darkness and light rages on, and that forgiving others is often the hardest choice to make. I've seen so many people talk about how it only hurts you when you hold on to resentments, it's almost cliché. I only can speak from my own experience, and say that to be able to fully participate in the joy that came with Brian coming back to us, my heart had to be free of that weight. Again, I thank God for giving that gift to me. What a beautiful miracle that is on its own accord.

22

Gratitude

The following is a post on our CaringBridge site that I wrote on May 26, 2012.

 I was watching Oprah (yes, Oprah) and she had on T. D. Jakes, a famous television minister. I'd probably seen him while flipping through channels, but never actually heard him speak. A clip from the show featured him preaching about the miracle of the loaves and fishes. I will paraphrase his interpretation, you can find the whole thing on the Oprah website if you want. He said two things that hit home to me.

First, was that during this miracle they collected the couple of fish and loaf of bread and then they blessed it. He stopped and made a beautiful point that they blessed what was inadequate, what was not enough. Following this, God blessed the crowd with so much that there were baskets and baskets left over after all had eaten their fill.

Thank God for what you have, even if it's not enough. As I heard him speak this, my mind immediately went to the dark days of December and January. David and my faith led us to practice this tenant without even realizing we were doing it. We thanked God for our broken and "hopeless" boy. We thanked him for giving us a peaceful place at the hospice for Brian to depart from us. We thanked him for what was nowhere near enough.

Pastor Jakes also talked about this miracle in that Jesus took the bread and broke it, and then blessed it. That the miracle was in the breaking . . . and if you feel you are broken, look to see where God is about to bless you. We surely felt broken, and it's taken all this time for the pain to finally dull.

Now six months later, look at the abundance of blessing God has put into our lives. Not only did Ben recover and flourish (finishing fifth grade with all A's, Principal's Honor Roll, and becoming a Boy Scout) but our Brian has defied the odds, and continues to show me every day that God is *always* in control.

God wants us to thank him for what we have, and yet why is it so hard to do? We're so grateful Brian is walking again (with help/support) but . . . the other side is, he should be running around like he used to. Thank God for the walking! We are excited when we see him beginning to gain control over his emotions and behavior but . . . it's still hard seeing him more like the three year old Brian in patience and self-control. Thank God he's talking at all!

Always be thankful, always stop and see what you *have,* not what you lack. The more I contemplate this, the more I feel it's one of the biggest lessons I was meant to learn through this ordeal, and if I could actually get there, would probably lead to a pretty amazingly fulfilled life. So I'll keep working on it!

I think maybe it was taking me too long to get this out of my system because the other night, totally out of the blue, I turned on Joel Olsteen (another TV preacher . . . all of this being kind of odd because I don't normally go out seeking religion there). Anyway, he was preaching about people who have overcome any bad circumstance in life and that we all should remember, *no matter what horrible things happen to us, before any of that happened, God blessed us and loved us.*

So, your earthly circumstances may be horrific (brain injury) but so what? That doesn't beat out God's plan for your life. If God has something amazing in store for you, nothing that happens to you can alter it. Wow. I had to just stop and think, "What does God have in mind for Brian?" It must be incredible because he literally brought Brian from the brink in order to have this destiny be able to come true. It's a powerful image for me and it just went hand in hand with the first message.

Don't be a victim. Don't allow circumstances (intentional or accidental) to rule how you live your life. Can I control what happened to Brian? No. Can I control how I react to it, and how I view our life now? Absolutely. Can I still find joy and happiness and gratitude every day? I have to, and if I do, I truly believe the incredible blessings will continue to flow.

During the nearly year and a half since I wrote this post, the lessons I was hoping to share in it have resonated with me over and over again. I feel certain that no amount of progress in Brian would have been "enough" if we had not been grateful for where we had come from. So often we can all fall into the trap of seeing only what we lack, rather than what we have. It's a human experience, one that unfortunately plays on our fears and doubts.

I see the circumstances we are dealt in life are always an opportunity though. When we can allow ourselves to rise out of the everyday perceptions that color our attitude about whatever the situation may be (relationship problem, loss of a job, illness, or even death of loved ones) we can view any negative situation from a totally different perspective. We can find gratitude in even the worst of times.

I don't pretend to know how or why our souls encounter the things that we do while in these physical bodies. Do we choose the life we get? If so, our soul must know something we cannot usually see—the good that comes from the situations in human lives that seem so tragic. If life is random, I do know for sure we can choose how we want to live regardless of the circumstances. How different would our situations seem to us if we could simply say, "Thank you, God, for giving me this experience, because though I cannot see it now, it is happening for the good"?

I have one particular piece of scripture that I have loved over the years, Philippians 4:2:

 Rejoice in the Lord always, again I will say Rejoice. Let your gentleness be known to everyone. The Lord is near. Do not worry about anything, but in everything by prayer and supplication with thanksgiving let your requests be made known to God. And the peace of God, which surpasses all understanding, will guard your hearts and your minds in Christ Jesus.

It meant so much to me that David and I included it in our wedding, and I can remember the priest making the point that St. Paul wrote this particular message from a prison cell. A place where most would be bitter or frustrated, instead of expressing those emotions, he called on us to find our higher ideals. How little our human experience has really changed in these two thousand years. What a beautiful example to try to live by. Each day, I do my best to rejoice, be thankful, and then bask in the love and peace I feel when I can succeed in doing so.

It doesn't have to be complicated. It's as simple as the prayer Brian and Ben say each night: "Thank you, God, for my mom and dad and brother. Thank you for this day. Amen."

Epilogue

Many months after the accident, on a return trip to Statesboro, we drove right by that same cemetery we at one point expected would be Brian's final resting place. But this day we were just driving by it, no reason to pay it much attention. Except our Brian was in his car seat, talking and joking with Ben, and noticed it. "Hey, look at the gravestones," he said. He smiled, went back to laughing with his brother, and we kept driving. How can it be that the boy that should have been laid to rest in that place was instead in the back seat of the car with his brother? How, instead of never hearing his voice or seeing his eyes light up again, we could see and hear him so full of life, laughter, and love? It all comes down to this: God is real. He loves us so much. And he can do miracles you almost have to see to believe.

Acknowledgments

Our story is filled with individuals and groups who made such an enormous impact on our lives during this tragedy. We wish to thank everyone who prayed for us, offered us assistance in any way, and played a part in this miracle. The names listed below are in no particular order.

Jennifer Murkison, Tim and Stephanie Laffey, Bridget Laffey, Dennis Laffey, Jimmy and Elisabeth Murkison, April Schueths, Nathan Palmer, Becky Holmes, Jodi Middleton Kennedy, the Thompson family, the Murphree family, the Townsend family, the Huling family, Kate and Jamie Williams, Pittman Park United Methodist Church, Jonathan Smith, St. Matthew Catholic Church, Fr. John Lyons, Fr. Brett Brannen, Fr. Pat O'Brien, Fr. Tim McKeown, Pastor Rachel Butler Grier, Pastor Doug, the staff and volunteers of the Ronald McDonald House of the Coastal Empire, the nursing staff of the Memorial Pediatric ICU, Nancy Hester, the staff at the Coastal Georgia Center, Becky and Issa Daou, Frank D'Arcangelo, Lissa Leege, the Harvey family, the staff and faculty of Georgia Southern University, John Paletta, Katie Jasionowski, the staff of Ogeechee Area Hospice, Joel and Azure Rountree, the Hughes Family, Greg Bucci, Susan Manack, Todd Williford and the staff of Sallie Zetterower Elementary, Dr. Carla Branch, the Caplinger/Malcom family, Dr. Dan McGuire, Terri Williams, Terry Johnson, Cara Wilt and the entire staff of Evansdale Elementary, the Claussen family, the

Hatfield family, the Todd family, the White family, the Fritz family, the Tso family, the Wakeman family, the staff of Children's Healthcare of Atlanta Comprehensive Rehabilitation Unit and Day Rehab (especially Yvette Shepard), the physical, occupational, and speech therapists at CHOA North Druid Hills outpatient facility(especially Megan Carroll), Amanda Giger, Dr. Lissa Davis Tchernis, Dr. Cindy Schoell, Linda Wright, Barb Garvin and the Holy Cross Catholic church family, Rebecca Rose, Ms. Madeline, Ms. Elizabeth, Pastor Tommy Ferrell and the Briarlake Baptist Church family, the O'Brien family, the Carney family, Ms. Joanne Weber, Ms. Renaye Middlebrook, Dr. Michael Braz, Lori and DeWayne Grice, Niamh Matthews, Mary Brammar, Kristina Bonham, the staff at Statesboro Bulloch County Parks and Recreation, Cheri Rourk, and the medical staff at Rehabilitation Associates of Atlanta.

A special thanks to the staff of BookLogix, Lori Grice Photography, and Deborah Harvey Graphic Design for helping make this book a reality.

To our parents: Bud and Carole Laffey and Gene and Marilyn Murkison. All of your faith, support, and encouragement have made it possible to get where we are today.

And finally, to Kristen and Joe Ruhland, who dropped everything to be with us through the darkest night, and through the joys and light that followed. There are no words to express my gratitude, but I will never forget your sacrifices for us. You are the truest definition of the word friend.

About the Author

Ellen Murkison is a mom, a writer, an inspirational speaker, and enjoyed a long career in the field of higher education prior to becoming a full-time caregiver for her kids in 2011. She and her husband David have two children, Ben and Brian, and live in Georgia.

Visit her online at www.EllenMurkison.com.